The EU Paediatric Regulation

PHARMACEUTICALS POLICY AND LAW

Pharmaceuticals Policy and Law

Volume 11

Earlier published in this series

Vol.1. J.L. Valverde and G. Fracchia (Eds), Focus on Pharmaceutical Research

Vol.2. J.L. Valverde (Ed), The Problem of Herbal Medicines Legal Status

Vol.3. J.L. Valverde (Ed), The European Regulation on Orphan Medicinal Products

Vol.4. J.L. Valverde (Ed), Information Society in Pharmaceuticals

Vol.5. C. Huttin (Ed), Challenges for Pharmaceutical Policies in the 21st Century

Vol.6. J.L. Valverde and P. Weissenberg (Eds), The Challenges of the New EU Pharmaceutical Legislation

Vol.7. J.L. Valverde (Ed), Blood, Plasma and Plasma Proteins: A Unique Contribution to Modern Healthcare

Vol.8. J.L. Valverde (Ed), Responsibilities in the Efficient Use of Medicinal Products

Vol.9(1,2). J.L. Valverde (Ed), 2050: A Changing Europe. Demographic *Crisis* and Baby Friend Policies

Vol.9(3,4). J.L. Valverde (Ed), Key Issues in Pharmaceuticals Law

Vol.10. J.L. Valverde and D. Watters (Eds), Focus on Immunodeficiencies

The EU Paediatric Regulation

Pharmaceuticals Policy and Law
Volume 11, 2009

Editors

J.L. Valverde
University of Granada, Granada, Spain
and
A. Ceci
Consorzio per Valutazioni Biologiche e Farmacologiche, Pavia, Italy

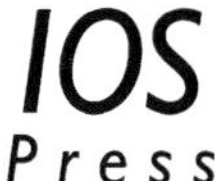

Amsterdam • Washington, DC • Tokyo

ISBN 978-1-58603-841-0
Library of Congress Control Number: 2008921406

Publisher
IOS Press
Nieuwe Hemweg 6B
1013 BG Amsterdam
The Netherlands
fax: +31 20 687 0019
e-mail: order@iospress.nl

Distributor in the UK and Ireland
Gazelle Books
Falcon House
Queen Square
Lancaster LA1 1RN
United Kingdom
fax: +44 1524 63232

Distributor in the USA and Canada
IOS Press, Inc.
4502 Rachael Manor Drive
Fairfax, VA 22032
USA
fax: +1 703 323 3668
e-mail: iosbooks@iospress.com

Distributor in Germany, Austria and Switzerland
IOS Press/LSL.de
Gerichtsweg 28
D-04103 Leipzig
Germany
fax: +49 341 995 4255

Distributor in Japan
Ohmsha, Ltd.
3-1 Kanda Nishiki-cho
Chiyoda-ku, Tokyo 101
Japan
fax: +81 3 3233 2426

Printed in the Netherlands

PHARMACEUTICALS POLICY AND LAW
Volume 11(1,2), 2009

CONTENTS

Pharmaceuticals Policy and Law 11 (2009) 1–2
DOI 10.3233/PPL-2009-0212
IOS Press

Editorial

The Regulation of Paediatric Medicines in the EU

The EU has been provided with a Regulation that promotes and regulates paediatric medicines.

Its gestation and negotiation in the inter-institutional legal triangle are an exact reflection of the glories and miseries of European construction. It is frequently said that EU legislation is made behind the backs of its citizens and imposed by the bureaucrats of Brussels. This cliché is as false as it is common, as confirmed by the negotiations of the Regulation on Paediatric Medicines.

The initiation of the preparation of the Regulation was made in response to the widespread demand of the scientific community, the health authorities and even of public opinion. The reasons why medicinal products need to be studied in children are clear: more than 50% of the medicines used to treat the children of Europe have not been tested; the paediatric population is a vulnerable group with developmental, physiological and psychological differences from adults; there are differences in pharmacokinetics and dynamics; growth and maturation processes affect them. And there is a general lack of information and appropriate pharmaceutical formulations. To overcome this lack, clinical trials have to be carried out on children, which, in turn, create serious scientific, legal and ethical problems. Specific protection should be defined for research performed on children, at all stages and ages. In order to address the concerns about trials in children, the EU Directive on clinical trials lays down specific requirements to protect children who take part in clinical trials in the EU. The Commission is developing guidelines to implement this Directive.

Once more, the European Medicines Agency (EMEA), in its function as the scientific organ of assessment and evaluation of medicinal products, prepared the scientific and technical foundations for the proposed legislation.

In 1997, the EMEA organised a round table of experts to discuss paediatric medicines. In 1998, the Commission supported the need for international discussion on the performance of clinical trials in children. An ICH guideline was therefore agreed, which has been in force since July 2002. This international agreement has been very important and has reaffirmed the need for and the possibility of advancing toward a global legal statute for medicinal products.

On 29 September 2004, the EU Commission released the first proposal for a Regulation on Medicinal Products for Paediatric Use. The Council of Health Ministers reached political agreement on 9 December 2005, and the European Parliament agreed it in a second reading on 1 June 2006. Thus it is difficult to understand why its publication was so delayed, it being such a sensitive subject from the social and health point of view.

It must be remembered that the European Regulation has followed the US initiative of 1977 and its consolidation in the *Paediatric Research Equity Act of 2003*. As a consequence of the US initiatives the response has been extremely positive.

Key measure included in the EU Regulation is the creation of the Paediatric Committee, within the European Medicines Agency whose principal task is to agree a Paediatric Investigational Plan (PIP) which results must be submitted at the time of the Marketing Authorisation (MA) application of new products as well as of authorised products where new indications, new pharmaceutical forms and new routes of administration are sought.

The requirements will not apply to generics. For drugs not yet authorised or still covered by a patent, the Regulation establishes rewards and incentives that include an extension (six months) of the patent. In case of Orphan Medicinal Products the incentive is represented by the extension of market exclusivity (12 years instead of 10).

In case of authorised products no longer covered by patent whose sponsor voluntarily apply for a MA in children, the Regulation provides a new type of marketing authorisation, the Paediatric Use Marketing Authorisation (PUMA) providing data protection for a ten-year period. To generate studies on off-patent products the Regulation includes the opportunity of accessing 'ad hoc' European funds for the research and development through the EU Research Framework Programmes.

Moreover, free scientific advice provided by the Agency is envisaged as an incentive to sponsors developing medicines for children. Likewise, one of the objectives of this proposal is to increase the information available on the use of medicines for children.

Paediatric patients deserve to have the same access as adults to effective medicines. Parents must be given sufficient information to give informed consent for their child to participate in pharmaceutical research. In the coming years we will observe more pre-clinical and clinical research, and a comparable debate has also started in Japan, Canada, Australia and other countries.

With this Regulation the EU has a solid regulatory framework for paediatric drug development that can promote a strong academic infrastructure for clinical research, and a greater competitiveness in the pharmaceutical industry. The subsidies established, although modest, will have the effect of providing legal certainty and a vision of European society and its institutions that will create a favourable climate for companies to foster pharmaceutical innovation in paediatric medicines and will permit an open and trustful dialogue between the key stakeholders for paediatric health care needs.

José Luis Valverde and Adriana Ceci
Co-editors

Pharmaceuticals Policy and Law 11 (2009) 3–9
DOI 10.3233/PPL-2009-0213
IOS Press

New paediatric research initiatives in the European Union

Fergal Donnelly
Scientific Officer, Health Biotechnology Unit, Health Directorate, Directorate General for Research and Technological Development, European Commission, Brussels, Belgium
E-mail: fergal.donnelly@ec.europa.eu

In contrast to the situation concerning adults, most medicines used to treat the children of Europe have not been tested on children and are not authorised for use in children. Therefore, the health and quality of life of children in the EU countries may suffer from a lack of testing and authorisation of medicines for their use. In particular, 46% of medicines prescribed to children in hospital are either unlicensed for their age group or, if they are, have been done so off-label [1]. Of the children who receive medication in hospital this figure rises to 67% [1], and in the context of intensive care up to 90% of paediatric medicines used are not licensed [2]. Although there may be concerns voiced about conducting trials in the paediatric population, this has to be balanced by the ethical concerns related to giving medicines to a population in which they have not been tested and therefore their effects, positive or negative, are unknown.

The European Parliament and Council Regulation on Medicinal Products for Paediatric Use [3] aims to improve the health of the children of Europe by increasing the research, development and authorisation of medicines for use in children, and as such represents a major breakthrough in paediatrics research. Its policy objectives are: to increase the development of medicines for use in children; to ensure that medicines used to treat children are subject to high quality research; to ensure that medicines used to treat children are appropriately authorised for use in children; to improve the information available on the use of medicines in children; and to achieve the above while avoiding unnecessary studies in children.

Ensuring that children have access to high-quality, effective and safe medicines, accompanied by high-quality information based on robust evidence, is crucial to giving children and their doctors the ability to make informed decisions about the treatment of disease and ensuring that the chosen medicines improve health. However, the diseases suffered by children often differ considerably from those suffered by adults, and the bodies of children tolerate drugs differently from those of adults.

The dose of a medicine to treat a childhood disease cannot always be extrapolated from the adult dose: medicinal products used in the paediatric population have never been specifically studied or authorised (licensed) for use in that age group. This leaves no alternative for the prescriber than to use products off-label – i.e. the use of a product authorised for adults (that is, products that have not been tested or authorised for paediatric use) – or the use of completely unauthorised products with the associated risks of inefficacy and/or adverse reactions (side effects). To remedy this state of affairs, new and established medicines will have to undergo research – including clinical trials in children – and pharmaceutical companies will have to obtain marketing authorisation based on the data generated. Medicines authorised for children will have to be marketed differently and clear and robust information about how and when to use the medicine will have to be available and accessible. The paediatric regulation proposes to address all of these factors through the specific policy objectives above. Within the context of the regulation, medicinal products can be broken down into three groups: products in development that have yet to be authorised; authorised products still covered by intellectual property rights (IPRs); and authorised products no longer covered by IPRs, i.e. off-patent.

The regulation contains a package of measures aimed at each of the above. Most apply to all, whereas others are specific to products falling into just one of the three groups listed above.

The first two of these categories involve requirements for new medicinal products and authorised medicines covered by a patent or a supplementary protection certificate (SPC). The purpose of this is to present the result of studies in children according to an agreed paediatric investigation plan at the time of marketing authorisation application or application for a new indication, novel dosage form or new route of administration.

A system of waivers will ensure that research in children is conducted only to meet the therapeutic needs of children, and a similar system of deferrals will ensure that research is carried out only when it is safe and ethical to do so. This will also ensure that the requirement for data in children will not block or delay the authorisation of medicines for other populations. For example, such studies in children may be funded by the European Commission (EC) and form part of a large scale project into a major subject or disease in paediatrics, where defining and testing potential remedies is but a part of a research and development programme.

Of major relevance to the Seventh Framework Programme (FP7) [4] is the third category of medicines, where there is no possibility of offering extended patent protection. Therefore, a new type of marketing authorisation is proposed – the Paediatric Use Marketing Authorisation (PUMA) – together with a study programme to fund or part-fund research into the paediatric use of off-patent medicines. PUMA is specifically for off-patent medicinal products developed exclusively for use in children, and provides a vehicle for awarding the incentive of data protection. This is an IPR that can be applied to off-patent medicines to stimulate innovation by allowing their use to treat new diseases and new populations. Of course, it is weaker than patent protection as competitors could carry out their own research and development programme on the same active substance if they judge the market to be big enough. Therefore, data protection is not a guarantee of market exclusivity.

In any case, an important argument against 're-awarding' market exclusivity to such products is that generics are already on the market and revoking their marketing authorisations is justified only if it is in the interest of public health, such as safety concerns. Quite simply, this means that market exclusivity is impossible in a multiproduct environment. Second, if – as has been suggested – the status of orphan medicine were to be awarded to such potentially new formulations, it would be contrary to the objective of promoting their general availability, since the orphan regulation aims to stimulate through incentives the development and authorisation of specific treatments for rare diseases. By definition, these are few in number, whereas the objective of this part of the regulation is for as many medicines on the EU market to be tested (other than generics) and authorised (including generics) for use in children and thereby to promote such availability. Therefore, data protection is considered to be the most practical option for all off-patent medicines for children even if the incentive is less when no child-specific formulation is required.

A study programme for off-patent medicines for children is now part of the FP74 and represents the other incentive anticipated by the regulation, i.e. "... Funds for research into medicinal products for the paediatric population shall be provided for in the Community budget in order to support studies relating to medicinal products or active substances not covered by a patent or a supplementary protection certificate. This is delivered through the Community Framework Programmes for Research, Technological Development and Demonstration Activities (Article 40)". It is based on a list of paediatric priorities for off-patent products devoid of commercial interest, drawn up by a group of experts in paediatrics at the European Medicines Agency (EMEA) and the Paediatric Committee (PDCO), for which studies would have to be publicly funded. Two selection criteria are applied, the first of which is conditions or disease states in terms of clinical seriousness and absence of therapeutically authorised alternatives, taking into particular account the need for neonatal treatment, where such needs are most acute. The second criterion is a demonstration of therapeutic interest from published clinical reviews, especially from previous clinical trials in children of the data, efficacy or safety of pharmacokinetics (PK). The final judgement on whether to fund research will depend on the combination of these two considerations.

The original version of this programme has been used for the Call for Proposals launched in 2007 for each of these classes by the Paediatric Committee. Overall, the proposals received as a result of this Call covered a broad range of ages listed as being high priority and some of the conditions listed. There was generally good coverage of malignant diseases, infectious diseases and neonatology, but somewhat limited attention given to a number of paediatric specialties, e.g. no proposals in ophthalmology, gastroenterology or psychiatry, and only one proposal in cardiovascular medicine. New EU Member States were significantly under-represented. Of these proposals, six were recommended to receive funding, of which three deal with oncology and one each with respiratory medicine, the needs of neonates and infectious diseases. Another Call for Proposals is proposed for September 2008.

1. General observations

Some products will need full development in at least one age group, whereas others need only a complement of information followed by regulatory assessment. The cost of developing a formulation is about €750,000. In Europe, the cost of development by academic centres would be about €200,000 for a PK study, €500,000 for dose-finding work and €1.7m for efficacy and safety studies. Therefore, the limit of the EC contribution to these projects has been set at €6m per project.

A figure of €30m for the first Call for Proposals was set aside as the EC contribution for this research activity. Similar amounts may be proposed for future Calls. Of course, this does not include any additional preclinical development that may be required. It should also be emphasised that the entry into force of the Good Clinical Practice (GCP) Directive (EC No. 2001/20) as of May 2004 will significantly increase the cost of clinical development, as GCP requirements are labour-intensive. The extent of this is unknown to date.

The list will be updated periodically to maintain up-to-date estimates of the products. A final list of priority products will be available from the EMEA when the next Call for Proposals is launched on 3 September 2008.

Paediatric oncology merits special consideration because nearly all children with cancer have already been enrolled in numerous studies that have been published. Furthermore, broadly discussing ‘oncology’ *per se* does not necessarily address matters of drug development in the field where a given product’s antineoplastic activity outweighs the condition itself and will determine the combination of such drugs studied. However, as with other conditions, the lack of PK data in younger age groups and the lack of paediatric formulations are pressing. The preparation of extemporaneous formulations of highly toxic oncology products requires additional precautions over and above those needed for other pharmaceutical entities and entails additional risks to those of extemporaneous paediatric preparations in general. The needs of children under three years of age will merit special consideration.

An added feature of the forthcoming Call for Proposals is that participating centres based in countries that are neither EU Member States nor associated countries (e.g. Albania, Croatia, the former Yugoslav Republic of Macedonia, Iceland, Israel, Liechtenstein, Montenegro, Norway, Serbia, Switzerland and Turkey) will be eligible to receive funding. This will enhance co-operation between European research centres and other top-quality organisations, e.g. in North America, for the benefit of children worldwide.

1.1. Other matters for consideration

Additional concerns that need to be addressed include the study of data that have been collected by cohorts and registries over decades to determine the long-term effects of medicines. In the future, childfriendly formulations for existing medicinal products need to be developed, and the needs of neonates and adolescents across the spectrum of all medicines and gender differences in the metabolism of medicines need to be considered.

2. Stakeholders

Children, their parents and their families are the ultimate stakeholders affected by the paediatric regulation. Currently, children are denied robustly tested, authorised medicines to meet their therapeutic needs; the main objective of the paediatric regulation is to improve the health of children by ensuring an adequate supply of such medicines. Their representatives are encouraged to participate in research proposals.

Healthcare professionals such as medical doctors, paediatricians and other specialists, pharmacists, nurses and researchers will want to provide their patients with effective, safe and high-quality products, rather than take personal legal liability for the effects of the untested, unauthorised medicines that they are bound to prescribe.

Health professionals are also involved in research into the effects of medicines in children and measures to increase research will influence those involved.

In much of the EU, national governments are ultimately responsible for healthcare, including medicines. They are responsible for promoting the health of their citizens and also have an economic interest in having a healthy population with low healthcare and social security needs who are able to work and generate wealth.

Other stakeholders are the authorities who regulate the pharmaceutical industry. More specifically they are responsible for the approval of clinical trials in Europe, the authorisation of medicines and manufacturing facilities, inspecting factories, laboratories, clinical trials and market authorisation holders, maintaining marketing authorisations and pharmacovigilance, which means monitoring the safety of marketed medicines, and taking action to increase benefit and reduce risk from them.

The pharmaceutical industry comprises large companies (a few that are predominantly based in the EU) and smaller companies (many more that are firmly based in the EU). Furthermore, the industry can be divided into the innovative industry, responsible for the discovery, research and development of innovative medicines, and the generics industry, which is responsible for limited research only but undertakes the manufacture of generic copies of off-patent innovative medicines.

Many generic pharmaceutical companies can be classified as small and medium-sized enterprises (SMEs) [5], as they have fewer than 250 employees, an annual turnover not exceeding €50m and a balance sheet not exceeding €43m. This sector is of special interest to the FP7 as they represent an important part of its client base. Another important member of this category is the contract research organisation (CRO). All potential SMEs are urged to register as such with the EMEA [6]. This will enable considerable savings to be made in the seeking of various degrees of scientific advice and inspection fees at the EMEA by reductions of up to 90% and the deferral of payments for such advice until after successful authorisation of products.

3. The main provisions for small and medium-sized enterprises

A variety of incentives have been established to assist SMEs: administrative and procedural assistance from the SME Office at the EMEA; fee reductions for scientific advice (90% fee reduction) and inspections; fee exemptions for certain administrative services (excluding parallel distribution); deferral of the fee payable for an application for marketing authorisation or related inspections; conditional fee exemption where scientific advice is followed and a marketing authorisation application is not successful; and assistance with translations of the product information documents submitted in the application for marketing authorisation.

A responsible and dedicated office has been established at the EMEA for the submission of requests for designation of SME status and to answer queries [6]. A comprehensive guide has been published giving further information [7].

4. Conclusion

Europe's children deserve the highest standards of research and ethical protection, and these initiatives are designed to provide this.

Based on the existing and considerable resources in the form of off-patent medicines, more research can now be initiated and outcomes can be directly brought 'from bench to bedside' in one of the first initiatives of its kind worldwide. This is already showing results in terms of a positive impact on the health and wellbeing of children, while at the same time boosting the innovative capacity of European health-related industries and businesses and promoting international collaboration.

Acknowledgement

This article was first published at: Donnelly F, New Paediatric Research Initiatives in the European Union, *European Paediatrics* **2**(1) (2008), 10–12. Reprinted with permission.

References

[1] S. Conroy, I. Choonara, P. Impicciatore et al., Survey of unlicensed and off-label drug use in paediatric wards in European countries, *Br Med J* **320** (2000), 79–82.

[2] M. Chalumeau, J.M. Tréluyer, B. Salanave et al., Off label and unlicensed drug use among French office based paediatricians, *Arch Dis Child* **83** (2001), 502–505.

[3] Regulation (EC) No. 1901/2006 of the European Parliament and of the Council of 12 December 2006 on medicinal products for paediatric use and amending Regulation (EEC) No. 1768/92, Directive 2001/20/EC, Directive 2001/83/EC and Regulation (EC) No 726/2004 (Text with EEA relevance) *Official Journal of the European Union*, L 378/1 27.12.2006.

[4] Decision No. 1982/2006/EC of the European Parliament and of the Council of 18 December 2006 concerning the Seventh Framework Programme of the European Community for Research, Technological Development and Demonstration Activities (2007–2013), *Official Journal of the European Union*, L 412/1, 30.12.2006.

[5] Commission Recommendation of 6 May 2003 concerning the definition of micro, small- and medium-sized enterprises (notified under document number C(2003) 1422), *Official Journal of the European Union*, 20.5.2003 L 124/36–41.

[6] http://www.emea.europa.eu/htms/human/presub/q47.htm.
[7] SME definition, User guide and model declaration, European Commission, EN NB-60-04-773-EN-C 92-894-7909-4.

Pharmaceuticals Policy and Law 11 (2009) 11–12
DOI 10.3233/PPL-2009-0214
IOS Press

TEDDY Network of Excellence: Monograph on paediatric medicines

Adriana Ceci
Consorzio per Valutazioni Biologiche e Farmacologiche, Pavia, Italy
E-mail: aceci@cvbf.net

TEDDY (Task-force in Europe for Drug Development for the Young) is a Network of Excellence funded under the Sixth EU Framework Programme for Research and Technological Development (FP6) whose mission is to promote the availability of safe and effective medicines for children in Europe by integrating existing expertise in order to stimulate further developments.

One of TEDDY main objectives is 'to build critical mass capacity by means of training and education activities, dissemination of information and development of guidelines'.

Thus, in accordance with its aims and to ensure the diffusion of results to a wide audience, TEDDY has chosen promotional and dissemination instruments (give-aways, posters, presentation CDs, exhibitions, thematic mailing lists) among which there is the publication of manuscripts in scientific journals.

This monograph, part of the activities TEDDY carried out to achieve its aim, constitutes of the following ten articles:

- "TEDDY NoE project in the framework of the EU Paediatric Regulation", presenting the TEDDY project and the results obtained in the first 3 years of activities.
- "The role of paediatric pharmacogenetic studies in Europe", exploring the current status, limitations and perspectives of pharmacogenomic and pharmacogenetic clinical research in the paediatric population.
- "TEDDY EPMD: a European Paediatric Medicines Database", presenting TEDDY EPMD and the analysis carried out to discuss the 'state of the art' of paediatric medicines licensed by European Medicines Agency (EMEA) in its first 12 years of activities.
- "Off-label and unlicensed use of medicines for children", referring on the results of a survey carried out to reach a common definition of the terms off-label and unlicensed use of medicines in children to favour the use of a European official regulatory terminology and facilitate pharmaco-epidemiological research.
- "Paediatric status and off-label use of drugs in children in Italy, United Kingdom and the Netherlands", comparing the extent of the off-label use in Italy, United Kingdom and The Netherlands.

- "Recommendation for Drug Development for Children", identifying the unmet therapeutic needs for the development and use of medicinal products in male/female children.
- "Clinical trials for paediatric medicines in Europe", evaluating the status of paediatric clinical trials performed for drugs to be used in children to verify their methodology and their compliance with the Note for Guidance ICH Topic E11.
- "Activity of Ethics Committees in Europe on issues related to clinical trials in paediatrics: results of a survey", referring on the results of a survey carried out to examine the measures enforced by Member States to implement the EU Clinical Trials Directive and other ethical norms relevant for clinical research in paediatrics.
- "Adverse Drug Reactions (ADRs) reporting in children", studying the frequency and the type of ADR reporting in children.
- "Availability of medicines for rare diseases in EU Countries", referring on the results of a questionnaire aimed at collecting information on orphan medicinal products availability, administered to twelve Member States.

Pharmaceuticals Policy and Law 11 (2009) 13–21
DOI 10.3233/PPL-2009-0206
IOS Press

TEDDY NoE project in the framework of the EU Paediatric Regulation

A. Ceci[a,*], P. Baiardi[a], F. Bonifazi[b], C. Giaquinto[c], M.J. Mellado Peña[d], P. Mincarone[b], A. Nicolosi[e], M. Sturkenboom[f] and I. Wong[g]
[a]*Consorzio per Valutazioni Biologiche e Farmacologiche, Pavia, Italy*
[b]*I.RI.D.I.A. srl, Health Care Engineering, Bari, Italy*
[c]*Department of Paediatrics, University of Padova, Padova, Italy*
[d]*Department of Paediatrics, Hospital Carlos III, Madrid, Spain*
[e]*Italian Embassy in Belgium, Brussels, Belgium*
[f]*Pharmacoepidemiology Unit, Departments of Medical Informatics and Epidemiology & Biostatistics, Erasmus University Medical Center, Rotterdam, The Netherlands*
[g]*Centre for Paediatric Pharmacy Research, The School of Pharmacy and Institute, Contro Nazionale delle Ricerche-Tecnologie Biomediche, Milan, Italy*

The lack of good quality medicines with formulations tailored for children and supported by properly conducted clinical trials or high level clinical evidence is a longstanding problem in Europe and worldwide.

The adoption of the new Paediatric Regulation (Reg. 1901/2006/EC), which forces pharmaceutical industries to conduct a paediatric investigation plan (PIP), is expected to increase the availability of properly tested and authorised medicines for paediatric use.

In this framework, the Task-force in Europe for Drug Development for the Young (TEDDY) Network of Excellence was established in 2005 to promote cooperation among researchers and other important stakeholders (regulatory authorities, professionals, patients and consumers) in order to optimise the paediatric use of current drugs and promote the development of new drugs for children, thus actively supporting the implementation of the European Paediatric Regulation.

Keywords: TEDDY, paediatric medicine, FP6 project, Network of Excellence, Paediatric Regulation, Europe

1. Introduction

The lack of good quality medicines with formulations tailored for children and supported by properly conducted clinical trials or high level clinical evidence is a longstanding problem in Europe and worldwide. Existing drugs are often used off-label and lack child safety and efficacy data.

This gap is rooted, on the one hand, in the complexity of scientific and ethical issues linked to the design and execution of clinical trials involving children, and on the other hand, on a perception of poor profitability which seems to prevent pharmaceutical

*Corresponding author: Adriana Ceci, Consorzio per Valutazioni Biologiche e Farmacologiche, Via Palestro, 26 – 27100 Pavia, Italy. Tel.: +39 0382 25075; Fax: +39 0382 536544; E-mail: aceci@cvbf.net.

companies from investing significantly in this sector. However, along with other age groups, also children should benefit from breakthroughs in genomics, biotechnology, pharmacology and therapeutics.

The adoption of the new Paediatric Regulation (Reg. 1901/2006/EC), which forces pharmaceutical industries to conduct a paediatric investigation plan (PIP), is expected to increase the availability of properly tested and authorised medicines for paediatric use.

In this framework, the Task-force in Europe for Drug Development for the Young (TEDDY) Network of Excellence (NoE) was established in 2005 to promote cooperation among researchers and other important stakeholders (regulatory authorities, professionals, patients and consumers) in order to optimise the paediatric use of current drugs and promote the development of new drugs for children, thus actively supporting the implementation of the European Paediatric Regulation.

2. The Task-force in Europe for Drug Development for the Young (TEDDY)

TEDDY is a Network of Excellence funded under the Sixth EU Framework Programme for Research and Technological Development (FP6) whose overall aim is to promote the availability of safe and effective medicines for children in Europe by integrating existing expertise and good practices, as well as stimulating further developments. The project started in June 2005 and is expected to run until 2010. Uniting 19 Partners from 10 EU Countries plus Israel (Table 1), it works closely with the European Commission, especially the Directorate-General for Research.

TEDDY represents a new focus in the paediatric pharmaceutical research, it differs from a scientific society, a network for developing research or trials, or a consultative regulatory body. Its ambition is to support existing paediatric networks, societies and regulatory bodies to undertake novel initiatives, including those in areas which such undertakings would not be feasible without a supportive action.

To fulfil its goals, TEDDY set up a very complex and hard to coordinate structure incorporating 7 Objectives (Table 2) and 12 WorkPackages (WPs) (Table 3). Life science related topics as pharmacogenomics, developmental and gender characteristics, and other paediatric medicines related topics (drugs availability, paediatric prescription and ADRs, therapeutic needs and research priorities) were included in the Network's activities and participants were asked to collaborate in a durable integration of their research capacities and knowledge.

3. TEDDY activities and results

TEDDY activities concentrated on life science and paediatric medicines related topics, with the purpose of stimulating the interaction of paediatric research groups

Table 1
TEDDY NoE partners

No	Participant	Country
1	Consorzio per Valutazioni Biologiche e Farmacologiche (Coordinator)	Italy
2	Azienda Ospedaliera di Padova	Italy
3	University College London	United Kingdom
4	Universiteit Leiden	The Netherlands
5	Consiglio Nazionale delle Ricerche – Istituto di Tecnologie Biomediche	Italy
6	Erasmus University Medical Cent	The Netherlands
7	Istituto Superiore di Sanita'	Italy
8	Romanian Angel Appeal	Romania
9	Linköpings Universitet	Sweden
10	Institut National De La Sante et Recherche Medicale	France
11	Medical Research Council Clinical Trials Unit	United Kingdom
12	Hospital Carlos III	Spain
13	Universite de Liége	Belgium
14	Institute of Physiology, Academy of Sciences, Lab. of Neurophysiology of Memory	Czech Republic
15	Technion – Israel Institute of Technology	Israel
16	Charité – Universitätsmedizin Berlin	Germany
17	Tecnofarmaci – Società Consortile per Azioni – per lo Sviluppo della Ricerca Farmaceutica	Italy
18	School of Pharmacy	United Kingdom
19	I.RI.D.I.A. S.r.L.	Italy

Table 2
TEDDY objectives

Objective 1	To establish a rationale for the safe and efficacious use of medicines in male/female children based on an understanding of developmental biology, pharmacogenetics and pharmacogenomics
Objective 2	To identify unmet needs for the development and use of medicinal products and orphan drugs in male/female children
Objective 3	To develop, validate and harmonise pre-clinical and clinical methods for assessing the safety and efficacy of both available and new drugs in male/female children.
Objective 4	To explore, validate and consolidate available information on medicine use in male/female children to support a harmonised, integrated and reliable European database (or system of databases)
Objective 5	To increase awareness of, and to contribute to the debate on, ethical issues arising from a) paediatric drug research and use, including off-label and unlicensed use, and b) the extended use of biotechnology for diagnostic and therapeutic purposes
Objective 6	To encourage the development of new drugs by bringing together industry and other relevant stakeholders, optimising paediatric formulations and providing labelling recommendations for available drugs
Objective 7	To build a critical mass capacity in Europe for the safe and efficacious use of medicines in male/female children, by means of training and education activities, dissemination of information and development of guidelines

on a multinational level and participating in initiatives proposed by the European Institutions to implement the new Paediatric Regulation.

The Network interacts and cooperates with the EMEA and the European Commission also by participating in public consultations on regulatory documents, providing

Table 3
WorkPackages list

No.	WorkPackage
1	Pharmacoepidemiology
2	Facilitation of the advancement of genomics and paediatric pharmacogenetic studies
3	Methodology of clinical studies in paediatrics
4	Addressing key therapeutic questions in children
5	Rare diseases
6	Postmarketing studies applied to paediatric medicine
7	Ethics
8	Paediatric Drug databases
9	Communication, Information & Learning
10	Management of the network
11	Collaboration with other initiatives and organisation
12	Gender issues in drug evaluation

Table 4
Networks and Paediatric Scientific Societies with stable collaboration with TEDDY

Networks
Paediatric European Network for the treatment of AIDS (PENTA)
Paediatric Rheumatology INternational Trials Organisation (PRINTO)
Relating Expectations and needs to the Participation and Empowerment of children in Clinical Trials (RESPECT)
European Clinical Research Infrastructures Network (ECRIN)
Priority Medicines For Children (ERA-NET PRIOMEDCHILD)
Early detection of adverse drug events by integrative mining of clinical records and biomedical knowledge (ALERT)
Paediatric Scientific Societies
SIOP Europe
European Paediatric Cardiology Association (AEPC)
European Society for P. Endocrinology (ESPE)
European Society for P. Infectious Diseases (ESPID)
European Respiratory Society (ERS)
SI per le Malattie Respiratorie Infantili (SIMRI)
European Society of Paediatric Gastroenterology, Hepatology and Nutrition (ESPGHAN)
Committee on Gastroenterology of the ESPGHAN
Società Italiana di Pediatria (SIP)
Societé Francaise de Pediatrie

comments and suggestions. Moreover, TEDDY experts provide contributions on the documents released by the EMEA Paediatric Working Party (PEG) and Paediatric Committee (PDCO).

TEDDY also carries out actions devoted at enlarging the influence of the Network and at promoting specific networking and paediatric research. A positive outcome of these activities is demonstrated by the number of researchers and subjects that joined the Network, including dedicated paediatric Networks, Scientific Societies (Table 4), Professionals and Parents/Patients Associations, Regulatory Bodies representatives, Pharmaceutical Companies and SMEs, as well as by the new research proposals including TEDDY partnership and leadership.

The aim of this report is to provide a brief presentation of TEDDY state of art and main results.

3.1. WP1: Pharmacoepidemiology

Paediatric prescription databases are few in Europe and no common standardised methodology for the collection of data is currently adopted.

TEDDY characterised the contents and main features of 18 prescription databases from 10 EU Countries, thus enabling subsequent assessments of consistency and reliability for the purposes of paediatric research.

Moreover, reports and 4 publications were produced using 3 prescription databases [1,4,7–11,14–18,20]. Four additional European databases are joining the research. Currently prescription data on 5 million paediatric patients are available for common pharmacoepidemiological studies.

TEDDY experts also considered the differences by ATC, age and Countries in 244,267 ADRs reports [19].

Finally, a two-stage, web-based Delphi survey was conducted among experts in Europe to develop common definitions for unlicensed and off-label drug use in children. A final proposal was adopted after consultation with the European Medicines Agency (EMEA) and the definitions will be circulated within the scientific community and recommended to be adopted by relevant regulatory authorities [12].

3.2. WP2: Facilitation of the advancement of genomics and paediatric pharmacogenetic studies

Before TEDDY's establishment, initiatives in this field were not focused on paediatrics (e.g. ad hoc CHMP/EMEA Phamacogenomics Working Party – PgWP).

TEDDY performed a review of the focus of published academic paediatric research in EU [6], unravelling the urgent need for confirmatory research to enable translation of potential PGt findings into label recommendations.

Moreover, a survey was conducted to identify the available expertise and the commonly used methodology in PGx/PGt and a methodological initiative aimed at including paediatric PGx/PGt into the paediatric development process is still ongoing.

3.3. WP3: Methodology of clinical studies in paediatrics / WP4: Addressing key therapeutic questions in children / WP5: Rare diseases / WP8: Paediatric Drug databases

Before the entry into force of the Paediatric Regulation, no activities similar to those carried out by TEDDY existed in Europe.

TEDDY created the European Paediatric Medicine Database (EPMD) storing data on almost 600 medicines (centralised and decentralised) [3]. The database also provides the opportunity to make comparisons of drugs availability, minimum approved age, price and reimbursement system on selected groups of drugs and in selected Countries.

TEDDY experts also completed an assessment of the methodological aspects of the existing paediatric trials (both for regulatory submission and non-regulatory purposes) dealing with the medicines in the database. This study included a comparison between centralised/decentralised drugs, rate and type of trials for regulatory submission and non-regulatory purposes. An article is in preparation.

A position paper on the methodological requirements for conducting clinical trials in children is in preparation.

Proposals on priorities for paediatric research have been made based on the availability of paediatric data and according to the recommendations of the 12 TEDDY Therapeutic Experts Groups. An article with specific focus on paediatric oncology was published [13] and others are in preparation.

TEDDY also investigated the availability of and need for paediatric orphan drugs.

Finally, in addition to the information available from EUDRACT and EUDRAPHARM, TEDDY offers a compilation of relevant data to the EMEA and other stakeholders, which are not covered by the current systems.

3.4. WP7: Ethics

TEDDY demonstrated capacity in communicating with stakeholders, including with Ethics Committees, and in scoping out proposals with wider, international involvement. TEDDY endeavours to contribute with upcoming Institutional initiatives.

The Network's first initiative was to perform a survey investigating the ethical and legal contexts before and after the implementation of Directive 20/2001/EC and encompassing 27 European Countries [2]. This investigation anticipated other similar initiatives.

Moreover, a questionnaire was used to measure consensus on initiatives aimed at implementing the recently approved European Commission Recommendations and a 'consensus position paper' is in preparation to be submitted to the EU Regulatory Body.

Finally, public discussions have been promoted to integrate the new paediatric rule in the current ethical and scientific debate and to increase awareness on this sensitive topic.

3.5. WP12: Gender issues in drug evaluation

Despite the emphasis of the European Commission on the need to consider gender aspects in paediatric research, no initiatives had been undertaken in this field.

TEDDY completed a bibliographic research on gender related differences in the incidence and/or prevalence of specific diseases at childhood [5] and an evaluation of the influence of gender on drug utilisation and ADRs rate and type in selected drugs classes.

Moreover, researchers interested in the paediatric gender issues were identified and asked to collaborate in future FP7 funded initiatives.

4. Conclusions: The future of the TEDDY network

TEDDY history is quite parallel with the Paediatric Regulation approval and entering into force. Many of the main innovations included in the Paediatric Regulation were anticipated by and included in TEDDY plan of activities: paediatric databases implementation, pharmacoepidemiology, clinical trials methodology and ethics.

For this reason, one of TEDDY main commitment is to support EMEA initiatives and maintain formal links with the EMEA at different levels. EMEA representatives participated in and actively contributed to TEDDY 3 "open" meetings (held respectively in Brussels on November 7th 2005, in Paris on February 13th and 14th 2006, and in Brussels on November 19th and 20th 2007). Similar initiatives will be carried out also with National Regulatory Agencies and with the Heads of Medicines Agencies (HMA).

At research level, TEDDY is building up research networks for the development of paediatric medicinal products through its Partners, providing support to researchers and pharmaceutical companies.

Moreover, TEDDY will be part of the Network of Paediatric Networks to be set up at the EMEA level and of the European Network of Centres of PharmacoVigilance and PharmacoEpidemiology (ENCePP), a new EMEA project.

In the next few years, the NoE will devote every effort to spread its results also among the general population, including especially minors and their families, with the aim of increasing the sensibility towards the need to provide children with tailored-made medicines and to support research in paediatrics.

Acknowledgements

This report is part of the Task-force in Europe for Drug Development for the Young (TEDDY) Network of Excellence supported by the European Commission's Sixth Framework Program (Contract n. 0005216 LSHBCT-2005-005126).

References

[1] R. Ackers, M.L. Murray, F.M. Besag and I.C. Wong, Prioritizing children's medicines for research: a pharmacoepidemiological study of antiepileptic drugs, *Br J Clin* **63**(6) (2007 Jun), 689–697. Epub 2007 Jan 25.

[2] A. Altavilla, C. Giaquinto and A. Ceci, European survey on ethical and legal framework of clinical trials in paediatrics: results and perspectives, *J Int Biœthique* **19**(4) (2008), in press.

[3] A. Ceci, M. Felisi, P. Baiardi, F. Bonifazi, M. Catapano, C. Giaquinto, A. Nicolosi, M. Sturkenboom, A. Neubert and I. Wong, Medicines for children licensed by the European Medicines Agency (EMEA): the balance after 10 years, *Eur J Clin Pharmacol* **62**(11) (2006), 947–952.

[4] M. Felisi, P. Baiardi, K. Verhamme, F. Sen, A. Neubert, L. Cantarutti and A. Ceci, Paediatric status and off-label use of drugs in children (oral presentation). *11th Biannual ESDP Congress* (4–7 June 2008), Rotterdam (The Netherlands).

[5] I. Grosch-Woerner, K. Verhamme, B. Kagedal, K. Vlcek, O. Vajnerova, A. Vanrolleghem and M. Sturkenboom, Gender issues in paediatric medicine. Recommendations on gender issues in clinical research management, available from URL: http://www.teddyoung.org [accessed 16 September 2008].

[6] E.H. Krekels, J.N. van den Anker, P. Baiardi, M. Cella, K.Y. Cheng, D.M. Gibb, H. Green, A. Iolascon, E.M. Jacqz-Aigrain, C.A. Knibbe, G.W. Santen, R.H. van Schaik, D. Tibboel and O.E. Della Pasqua, Pharmacogenetics and paediatric drug development: issues and consequences to labelling and dosing recommendations, *Expert Opin Pharmacother* **8**(12) (2007), 1787–1800.

[7] A.F. Medina Claros, M.J. Mellado Peña and F. Baquero Artigao, Bases para el uso clínico de fármacos en niños. Situación actual de uso de farmacos pediatricos en España, *An Pediatr Contin* **6**(3) (2008), 187–190.

[8] M.L. Murray, A. Neubert, G. Picelli, M.C.J.M. Sturkenboom, K.M.C. Verhamme, A. Ceci, C. Giaquinto, A. Nicolosi and I.C.K. Wong, Drug Utilisation of Neuropsychiatric Drugs in Children: A Multinational Study within the TEDDY Project (poster), *23rd International Conference on Pharmacoepidemiology & Therapeutic Risk Management*, (19–22 August 2007), Quebec City (Canada).

[9] A. Neubert, M.L. Murray, M.C.J.M. Sturkenboom, K.M.C. Verhamme, C. Giaquinto, A. Nicolosi, A. Ceci, G. Picelli and I.C.K. Wong, Drug Utilisation of Analgesics and Anti-Inflammatory Drugs in Children: A Multinational Database Study within the TEDDY Project (poster), *23rd International Conference on Pharmacoepidemiology & Therapeutic Risk Management* (19–22 August 2007), Quebec City (Canada).

[10] A. Neubert, M. Murray, M. Sturkenboom, K. Verhamme, A. Nicolosi, C. Giaquinto, A. Ceci and I, Wong, Population-Based Databases for Paediatric Medicine Research in Europe: A TEDDY Appraisal (poster), *23rd International Conference on Pharmacoepidemiology & Therapeutic Risk Management* (19–22 August 2007), Quebec City (Canada).

[11] A. Neubert, M.C.J.M. Sturkenboom, M.L. Murray, K.M.C. Verhamme, A. Nicolosi, C. Giaquinto, A. Ceci and I.C. Wong, Databases for Paediatric Medicines Research in Europe – Assessment and Critical Appraisal, *Pharmacoepidemiol Drug Saf* **17**(12) (2008 Dec), 1155–1167.

[12] A. Neubert, A. Bonifazi, M. Catapano, M. Felisi, P. Baiardi, C. Giaquinto, C. Knibbe, M.C.J.M. Sturkenboom, M.A. Ghaleb, I.C.K. Wong and A. Ceci, Defining Off-label and Unlicensed Use of Medicines for Children: Results of a Delphi survey, *Pharmacol Res* **58**(5–6) (2008 Nov–Dec), 316–322.

[13] P. Paolucci, K. Pritchard Jones, M. del Carmen Cano Garcinuno, M. Catapano, A. Iolascon and A. Ceci, Challenges in prescribing drugs for children with cancer, *Lancet Oncol* **9**(2) (2008 Feb), 176–183.

[14] E.F. Sen and M.C.J.M. Sturkenboom, The TEDDY Network: Epidemiological Trends in Paediatric Drug Use in Europe, *EJHP* **6** (2007), 22–24.

[15] E.F. Sen, K. Verhamme, A. Neubert, C. Giaquinto and M. Sturkenboom, Respiratory drug use in children in the Netherlands, Italy and United Kingdom (oral presentation). *11th Biannual ESDP Congress* (4-7 June 2008), Rotterdam (The Netherlands).

[16] M.C.J.M. Sturkenboom, K.M.C. Verhamme, M.L. Murray, A. Neubert, I.C. Wong, D. Caudri, G. Picelli, C. Giaquinto, L.i Cantarutti, A. Nicolosi, P. Baiardi and A. Ceci, Drug use in children: cohort study in three European countries. *BMJ* **337**:a2245 (2008 Nov 24), doi:10.1136/bmj.a2245.

[17] M.C. Sturkenboom, K.M. Verhamme, M.L. Murray, A. Neubert, G. Picelli, C. Giaquinto, A. Nicolosi, I. Wong and A. Ceci, General Drug Utilization in Children – A Multinational Database Study in the TEDDY Project (poster). *23rd International Conference on Pharmacoepidemiology & Therapeutic Risk Management* (19–22 August 2007), Quebec City (Canada).

[18] M.C.J.M. Sturkenboom, K.M.C. Verhamme, D. Caudri, M.L. Murray, A. Neubert, G. Picelli, C. Giaquinto, A. Nicolosi, I. Wong and A. Ceci, Respiratory Drug Use in Children: A Multinational Database Study in the TEDDY Project (poster). *23rd International Conference on Pharmacoepidemiology & Therapeutic Risk Management* (19–22 August 2007), Quebec City (Canada).

[19] K.M.C. Verhamme, P.M. Elferink-Stinkens, M.L. Murray, A. Neubert, A. Nicolosi, I. Wong, A. Ceci, B.H.Ch. Stricker and M.C.J.M. Sturkenboom, Adverse Drug Reaction Reporting in Children – The

Teddy Project (poster). *23rd International Conference on Pharmacoepidemiology & Therapeutic Risk Management* (19–22 August 2007), Quebec City (Canada).

[20] K.M.C. Verhamme, M.L. Murray, A. Neubert, G. Picelli, C. Giaquinto, A. Nicolosi, I. Wong, A. Ceci, M.C.J.M. Sturkenboom, Cardiovascular Drug Use in Children – The Teddy Project (poster). *23rd International Conference on Pharmacoepidemiology & Therapeutic Risk Management* (19–22 August 2007), Quebec City (Canada).

Pharmaceuticals Policy and Law 11 (2009) 23–30
DOI 10.3233/PPL-2009-0203
IOS Press

The role of paediatric pharmacogenetic studies in Europe

E. Krekels[a], A. Ceci[b,*], A. Iolascon[c], S. Girotto[d] and O. Della Pasqua[a]
[a]*Leiden/Amsterdam Center for Drug Research, Leiden, The Netherlands*
[b]*Consorzio per Valutazioni Biologiche e Farmacologiche, Pavia, Italy*
[c]*Department of Biochemistry and Medical Biotechnologies, University Federico II of Naples, CEINGE-Advanced Biotechnologies, Naples, Italy*
[d]*Azienda Ospedaliera di Padova, Padova, Italy*

Pharmacogenetics is a newly emerging research area confronted with obvious scientific and ethical concerns not only from an academic and social perspective, but also on a regulatory level.

An overview of ongoing and planned pharmacogenetic studies is needed to evaluate the current status and focus of research and to appraise the alignment of research themes relative to the unmet medical needs of the paediatric population.

The objective of this review was to explore the current status, limitations and perspectives of pharmacogenomic and pharmacogenetic clinical research in the paediatric population from an academic, regulatory and industrial perspective.

Results show a rather equal distribution of activities across the different research categories throughout the world. More than 50% of the research activities are related to exploratory studies aimed at establishing the connection between a given genetic trait and the risk associated with a pathology or disease.

Based on this situation, we advocate for more translational and conformational studies. Moreover, there is a strong need to give appropriate attention to the methodological requirements for clinical research, which lack the scientific and statistical rigour and make study findings unsuitable for clinical purposes and often impossible to interpret.

Keywords: TEDDY, paediatric medicines, pharmacogenetics, paediatric clinical trials

1. Introduction

An overview of ongoing and planned pharmacogenetic studies is needed to evaluate the current status and focus of research. Moreover, it enables an appraisal of the alignment of research themes relative to the unmet medical needs of the paediatric population.

When setting up a methodology for collecting accurate information relevant to studies involving pharmacogenetic research in children in the EU, three major problems were identified:

*Corresponding author: Adriana Ceci, Consorzio per Valutazioni Biologiche e Farmacologiche, Via Palestro, 26 – 27100 Pavia, Italy. Tel.: +39 0382 25075; Fax +39 0382 536544; E-mail: aceci@cvbf.net.

- Protocol titles in clinical trial databases often do not reflect research details for secondary endpoints; furthermore these endpoints are not classified as keywords either. Only approved or ongoing studies are available;
- Current search engines within clinical trial databases do not capture experimental procedures that describe pharmacogenetic-related assessments;
- The accuracy of the data due to lack of consistency in the update upon completion of studies is limited.

Therefore, an alternative methodology based on research published in PUBMED was implemented to identify ongoing scientific activities in pharmacogenetics in children.

Pharmacogenetics is a newly emerging research area confronted with obvious scientific and ethical concerns not only from an academic and social perspective, but also on a regulatory level. We were interested in investigating how regulatory agencies were handling such concerns in order to obtain further insight into the regulatory requirements, according to which investigators and industry have to perform.

In this report, it is assumed that pharmacogenetic findings should ultimately lead to labelling claims and dosing recommendations, which is a matter for industry rather than academia. Based on this assumption, we have attempted to assess to what extent pharmacogenetic research is being performed in children under the sponsorship of or in collaboration with pharmaceutical industry.

2. Objective of the review

The objective of this review is to explore the current status, limitations and perspectives of pharmacogenomic and pharmacogenetic clinical research in the paediatric population from an academic, regulatory and industrial perspective.

A literature search was conducted to obtain an overview of the academic efforts in pharmacogenomic and pharmacogenetic studies in children over the past 10 years. Information from this search is being abstracted into an overview that compares the activities in the EU, USA, Japan and the rest of the world.

The regulatory standpoint on pharmacogenomics and pharmacogenetics can be drawn from the vast amount of guidelines and regulations made public by regulatory agencies in this matter. This is however no easy task. The position of the agencies on this matter and their intentions for the future are even harder to find out in public sources. Therefore a secondary source was used to obtain insight in the current regulatory environment regarding pharmacogenetic research.

Similar difficulties were identified to assess to what extent pharmaceutical industry is active in pharmacogenomics and pharmacogenetics in children given the current regulation. At present, there is no consolidated source of information on industry activities with enough detail to allow accurate estimates. This gap is probably due to proprietor and patent issues, which prevent public disclosure of information. Our first attempt to consolidate publicly available data was based on search engines through the websites of major pharmaceutical companies with portfolio and pipeline for paediatric indications.

3. Academic research efforts

3.1. Methodology

A search was conducted using the MeSH database of PUBMED to obtain an overview of the academic efforts in pharmacogenomic and pharmacogenetic studies in children over the past 10 years. In this search the following keywords were used:

- *Infant*. Definition: person 1 to 23 months of age. Includes the terms: 'Newborn', 'low birth weight', 'postmature' and 'premature';
- *Child*. Definition: person 6 to 12 years of age. Includes the term: 'Child, preschool', which includes persons between 2 to 5 years of age;
- *Adolescent*. Definition: person 13 to 18 years of age;
- *Paediatrics*. Definition: a medical specialty concerned with maintaining health and providing medical care to children from birth to adolescence. Includes the terms: 'neonatology' and 'perinatology';
- *Human Development*. Definition: Continuous sequential changes which occur in the physiological and psychological functions during the life-time of an individual. Includes the terms: 'adolescent development' and 'child development'.

These words were cross-referenced with:

- *Pharmacogenetics*. Definition: A branch of genetics which deals with the genetic variability in individual responses to drugs and drug metabolism. Includes the term: 'Toxicogenetics'
- *Polymorphism, genetic**. Definition: The regular and simultaneous occurrence in a single interbreeding population of two or more discontinuous genotypes. The concept includes differences in genotypes ranging in size from a single nucleotide site to large nucleotide sequences visible at a chromosomal level. Includes the terms: 'Polymorphism, Restriction Fragment Length', 'Polymorphism, Single Nucleotide' and 'Polymorphism, Single-Stranded Conformational'
- *Genotype**. Definition: The genetic constitution of the individual; the characterization of the genes. Includes the terms: 'Gene dosage', 'Genetic Predisposition to Disease', 'Haplotypes', 'Heterozygote', and 'Homozygote'.
- *Pharmacokinetics*. Definition: Dynamic and kinetic mechanisms of exogenous chemical and drug absorption; biological transport; tissue distribution; biotransformation; elimination; and toxicology as a function of dosage, and rate of metabolism. It includes toxicokinetics, the pharmacokinetic mechanism of the

toxic effects of a substance. Includes the terms: 'Area Under Curve', 'Biological Availability', 'Biotransformation', 'Metabolic Clearance Rate', 'Metabolic Detoxication', 'Therapeutic Equivalency', and 'Tissue Distribution'.

- *AND Cytochrome P450 enzyme system.* Definition: A superfamily of hundreds of closely related hemeproteins found throughout the phylogenetic spectrum, from animals, plants, fungi, to bacteria. They include numerous complex monooxygenases. In animals, these P-450 enzymes serve two major functions: (1) biosynthesis of steroids, fatty acids, and bile acids; (2) metabolism of endogenous and a wide variety of exogenous substrates, such as toxins and drugs. They are classified, according to their sequence similarities rather than functions, into CYP gene families (>40% homology) and subfamilies (>59% homology). For example, enzymes from the CYP1, CYP2, and CYP3 gene families are responsible for most drug metabolism. Includes the terms: 'Aryl Hydrocarbon Hydroxylases', 'Aniline Hydroxylase', 'Benzopyrene Hydroxylase', 'Cytochrome P-450 CYP1A1', 'Cytochrome P-450 CYP1A2', 'Cytochrome P-450 CYP2B1', 'Cytochrome P-450 CYP2D6', 'Cytochrome P-450 CYP2E1', 'Cytochrome P-450 CYP3A', 'Camphor 5-Monooxygenase', 'Steroid Hydroxylases', '25-Hydroxyvitamin D3 1-alpha-Hydroxylase', 'Aldosterone Synthase', 'Aromatase', 'Cholesterol 7-alpha-Hydroxylase', 'Cholesterol Side-Chain Cleavage Enzyme', 'Steroid 11-beta-Hydroxylase', 'Steroid 12-alpha-Hydroxylase', 'Steroid 16-alpha-Hydroxylase', 'Steroid 17-alpha-Hydroxylase', and 'Steroid 21-Hydroxylase'.

To reduce the number of hits, the terms indicated with an asterisk (*) were set to the 'Restrict Search to Major Topic headings only' mode in the MeSH database.

A database was set up from articles on research in children that were published between January 1997 and December 2006. The selected articles were reports on heritable genetic changes and polymorphisms (also in mRNA). However, articles on somatic changes (for instance, genetic changes in tumour cells) were excluded at screening. Only original articles and reports were included in the data abstraction phase. Review articles, case reports, letters, and articles without abstract or without abstract in English were excluded from this evaluation.

Cross-referencing the aforementioned words resulted in articles on topics that are broader then pharmacogenomics and pharmacogenetics alone. The obtained articles were on general genetic research. During the literature search it became apparent that substantial efforts are allocated to genetic-based research in the paediatric population. However, the vast majority of this activity was of an exploratory nature, yielding limited information or knowledge that can be used or translated into medical practice.

To quantitatively assess resource allocation, the selected publications were grouped into the following categories based on the main focus of the reported investigation:

- *Sequence* (*S*): investigation of the genetic changes that occur in a certain disease.
- *Frequency* (*F*): investigation of how often a given gene/allele occurs in the population.

Table 1
The absolute amount of articles obtained in total for each geographical area and for each individual category

Area	Total	S	F	Pn	C	Ps	R	D	Py	Pa
EU	356	23	4	233	19	33	11	12	75	10
US	160	7	5	98	15	10	8	4	38	8
Japan	74	10	1	40	1	8	0	3	18	4
RoW	262	17	24	172	16	34	6	6	28	9

- *Predisposition* (*Pn*): investigation of the correlation between genetic traits and the probability or susceptibility for a given pathology or disease. The difference between 'Sequence' and 'Predisposition' is that the former involves only patients, whilst the latter includes affected and unaffected children in the population under investigation.
- *Clinical outcome* (*C*): investigation of the influence of a given genetic trait on the clinical outcome of a disease, on the event-free-survival or on the risk of relapse.
- *Prognosis* (*Ps*): investigation of the effect of a given genetic trait on disease progression, disease severity or risk of complications.
- *Risk* (*R*): investigation of the risk of adverse drug reactions (ADRs) associated with a specific genetic trait.
- *Diagnosis* (*D*): investigation of which genetic traits can be used to diagnose a disease.
- *Physiology* (*Py*): investigation of genotype/phenotype correlations, the role of genetic traits in drug metabolism, the role of genetic traits in pathology or investigation of the timing of gene activation (change in expression profile between child and adult).
- *Pharmacology* (*Pa*): investigation of the effect a genetic trait on drug response, drug resistance or target activation.

It is important to note that it is possible for an article to be in two or more categories. Four separate databases were created to compare the research activities in the EU with the USA, Japan and the rest of the world (RoW). Data were tabulated in ExcelTM (Microsoft Office) and summarised graphically as pie-charts.

4. Results and discussion

In February 2007 the database contained approximately 850 articles (Table 1).

The results of the study are presented in Fig. 1.

The pie-charts show a rather equal distribution of activities across the different research categories throughout the world. More than 50% of the research activities are related to predisposition, i.e. exploratory studies aimed at establishing the connection between a given genetic trait and the risk associated with a pathology or disease. A criticism to this type of exploratory work is that the majority of the

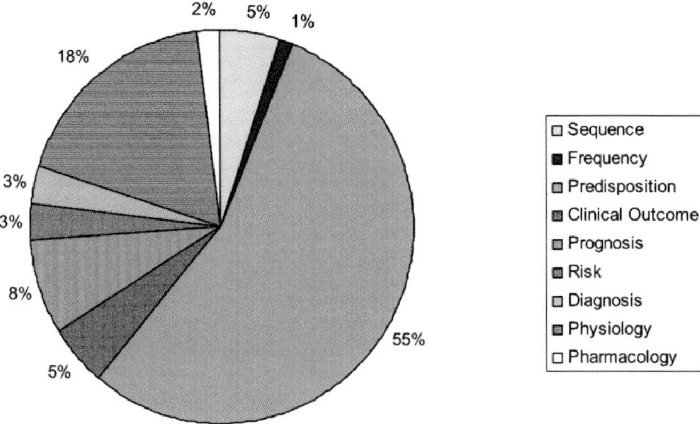

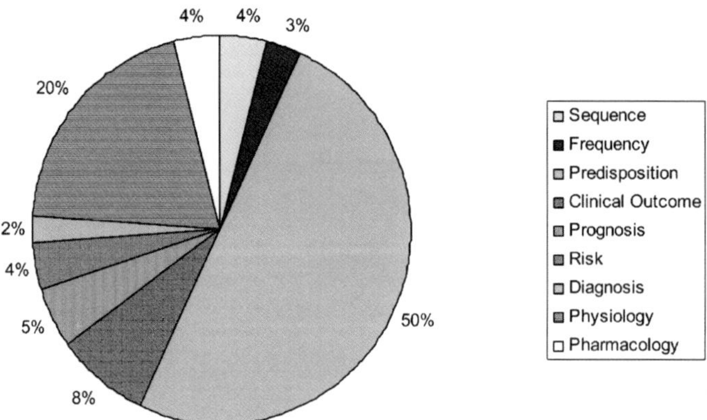

Fig. 1. Main focus of investigation of published research.

data captured during the study does not provide insight into mechanisms of diseases or drug action. Furthermore, it cannot be used to improve medical practice or support therapeutic solutions. The same limitation is observed for research activities in the categories 'Sequence', 'Frequency' and for most of the studies in the categories 'Clinical Outcome', 'Prognosis' and 'Risk'.

Research in the categories 'Physiology' and 'Pharmacology' is generally of a translational nature, yielding results that do give insight into mechanisms of disease, drug action or toxicity. Information obtained in these studies can be used to identify therapeutic targets or to establish labelling claims and dosing recommendations,

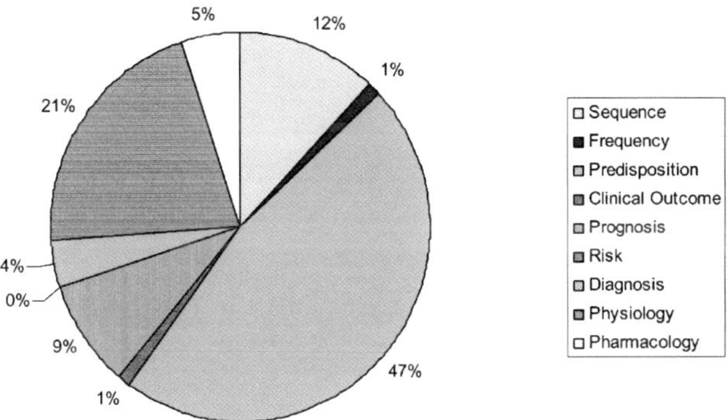

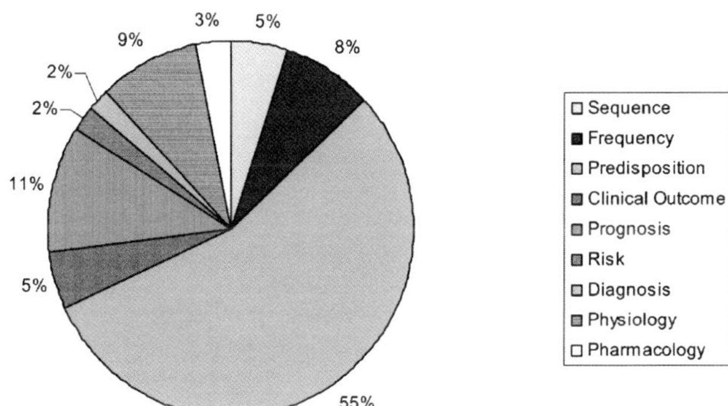

Fig. 1, continued.

which may eventually lead to therapeutic solutions and improvement of medical practice.

We realise that exploratory research is needed in order to proceed to translational investigations. However, the scientific output from contributing organisations and research institutes suggest that these investigations often stop when any connection between a genetic trait and disease, clinical outcome, disease progression or risk have been established. Findings also suggest that subsequent translational research remains neglected.

Based on the situation described above, we advocate for more translational and conformational studies. Moreover, we strongly feel the need to demand appropriate attention to the methodological requirements for clinical research, which lack the scientific and statistical rigour and make study findings unsuitable for clinical purposes and often impossible to interpret.

Acknowledgements

This report is part of the Task-force in Europe for Drug Development for the Young (TEDDY) Network of Excellence supported by the European Commission's Sixth Framework Program (Contract n. 0005216 LSHBCT- 2005-005126).

References

[1] M. Benzinou, A. Walley, S. Lobbens, M.A. Charles, B. Jouret, F. Fumeron, B. Balkau, D. Meyre and P. Froguel, Bardet-Biedl syndrome gene variants are associated with both childhood and adult common obesity in French Caucasians, *Diabetes* **55**(10) (2006 Oct), 2876–2882.

[2] Ch. Hartel, D. Finas, P. Ahrens, E. Kattner, T. Schaible, D. Muller, H. Segerer, K. Albrecht, J. Moller, K. Diedrich and W. Gopel, Genetic Factors in Neonatology Study Group, Polymorphisms of genes involved in innate immunity: association with preterm delivery, *Mol Hum Reprod* **10**(12) (2004 Dec), 911–915. Epub 2004 Oct 29.

[3] D.L. Jack, J. Cole, S.C. Naylor, R. Borrow, E.B. Kaczmarski, N.J. Klein and R.C. Read, Genetic polymorphism of the binding domain of surfactant protein-A2 increases susceptibility to meningococcal disease, *Clin Infect Dis* **43**(11) (2006 Dec 1), 1426–1433. Epub 2006 Oct 31.

[4] R. Marttila, R. Haataja, M. Ramet, M.L. Pokela, O. Tammela and M. Hallman, Surfactant protein A gene locus and respiratory distress syndrome in Finnish premature twin pairs, *Ann Med* **35**(5) (2003), 344–352.

[5] C. Modesto, A. Patino-Garcia, E. Sotillo-Pineiro, J. Merino, J. Garcia-Consuegra, R. Merino, M.J. Rua, L. Sierrasesumaga and C. Arnal, TNF-alpha promoter gene polymorphisms in Spanish children with persistent oligoarticular and systemic-onset juvenile idiopathic arthritis, *Scand J Rheumatol* **34**(6) (2005 Nov–Dec), 451–454.

[6] J. Svahn, M. Capasso, M. Lanciotti, A. Marrone, R. Haupt, A. Bacigalupo, C. Pongiglione, L. Boschetto, D. Longoni, M. Pillon, A. Pistorio, P. Di Michele, A.P. Iori, M. Calvillo, A. Locasciulli, G. Menna, R. Riccardi, U. Ramenghi, C. Dufour and A. Iolascon, The polymorphisms -318C>T in the promoter and 49A>G in exon 1 of CTLA4 and the risk of aplastic anemia in a Caucasian population, *Bone Marrow Transplant* **35**(Suppl 1) (2005 Mar), S89–S92.

[7] A. Treszl, I. Kocsis, M. Szathmari, A. Schuler, E. Heninger, T. Tulassay and B. Vasarhelyi, Genetic variants of TNF-[FC12]a, IL-1beta, IL-4 receptor [FC12]a-chain, IL-6 and IL-10 genes are not risk factors for sepsis in low-birth-weight infants, *Biol Neonate* **83**(4) (2003), 241–245.

Pharmaceuticals Policy and Law 11 (2009) 31–39
DOI 10.3233/PPL-2009-0211
IOS Press

TEDDY EPMD: A European Paediatric Medicines Database

M. Felisi[a], R. Padula[a], F. Bartoloni[b], I. Grosch-Wörner[c], B. Kagedal[d], M.J. Mellado Peña[e], J. Parry[f], A. Stuchlik[g], K. Verhamme[h] and A. Ceci[a,*]
[a]*Consorzio per Valutazioni Biologiche e Farmacologiche, Pavia, Italy*
[b]*I.RI.D.I.A. srl, Health Care Engineering, Bari, Italy*
[c]*Charité Universitätsmedizin Berlin, Berlin, Germany*
[d]*Department of Clinical Pharmacology, Linkopings Universitet, Linkopings, Sweden*
[e]*Department of Paediatrics, Hospital Carlos III, Madrid, Spain*
[f]*Romanian Angel Appeal, Budapest, Romania*
[g]*Department of Neurophysiology of Memory and Computational Neuroscience, Institute of Physiology, Academy of Sciences, Prague, Czech Republic*
[h]*Pharmacoepidemiology Unit, Departments of Medical Informatics and Epidemiology & Biostatistics, Erasmus University Medical Center, Rotterdam, The Netherlands*

In line with European initiatives, TEDDY set up a new database, the European Paediatric Medicines Database, with the aim of creating a harmonised, integrated and reliable pan-European source of information.

The data stored in the Database were the basis for examining the ‘state of the art’ of paediatric medicines licensed by the European Medicines Agency between October 1995 and December 2007.

The results of the study show that 33% of medicinal products approved by the European Medicines Agency are intended for the paediatric population, and that this percentage has remained more or less constant in the 12 years of activity of the Agency.

This trend is expected to increase rapidly in the future as a result of the adoption of the Paediatric Regulation.

Nevertheless, it is essential that information on medicinal products for paediatric use are made publicly accessible and data should be verified and controllable. The European Medicines Agency has recently made public many information on medicines authorised in EU through the EudraPharm database.

The TEDDY European Paediatric Medicines Database grants access also to information related to paediatric medicines, some of which are not available elsewhere.

We deem this aspect a useful service to end users and a valid support to Regulatory Authorities.

Keywords: TEDDY, paediatric medicines, EPMD, database

1. Introduction

The recently adopted European Paediatric Regulation [6] measures are devoted to assuring safe, effective and high quality drugs for children. In this context, innovative

*Corresponding author: Adriana Ceci, Consorzio per Valutazioni Biologiche e Farmacologiche, Via Palestro, 26–27100 Pavia, Italy. Tel.: +39 0382 25075; Fax +39 0382 536544; E-mail: aceci@cvbf.net.

drugs play a crucial role: children should be able to benefit from advances in modern therapies as well as adults.

In line with the European initiatives, TEDDY set up a new database, the European Paediatric Medicines Database (EPMD), with the aim of creating a harmonised, integrated and reliable pan-European source of information on innovative drugs and ultimately support further regulatory and legislative actions.

The data stored in the EPMD were the basis for discussing the 'state of the art' of paediatric medicines licensed by the European Medicines Agency (EMEA) in its first 12 years of activities and evaluating the characteristics of the medicines licensed for use in children by EMEA in the period October 1995 – December 2007.

2. The European Paediatric Medicines Database

The EPMD is a databank of innovative medicinal products for the paediatric population.

The objectives that TEDDY aims to achieve with this new instrument are to create a unique source of information, to support the transparency of the information concerning the innovative drugs currently used in children, to identify therapeutic areas uncovered by innovative drug treatments for children, and to provide health professionals, paediatricians, institutional bodies, companies, patients' associations, parents and children with appropriate information concerning the rational use of paediatric medicines.

The Database grants access to a drug library using a drug search engine that can be easily consulted.

The information collected in the EPMD can be grouped into 6 sections:

- General information (Table 1).
- Disease classification (Table 2).
- Therapeutic indication and prescription details (Table 3).
- Developmental status (Table 4).
- Medicinal products information (Table 5).
- Post-marketing modification of the medicinal product (Table 6):
  * MA variation.
  * Withdrawal.
  * Safety alert.

3. Paediatric drugs available for children

The main goal in the pharmaceutical field is to guarantee that efficacious, high quality and safe medicines are available to European citizens, regardless of income

Table 1
General information

Tradename	Commercial name given to the medicinal product
Active substance	International Nonproprietary Name (INN) or Common Name of substance carrying out the pharmacological action. Each INN is a unique name that is globally recognized. A nonproprietary name is also known as a generic name
ATC code	In the Anatomical Therapeutic Chemical classification code, drugs are classified in groups at 5 different levels:
Procedure of authorisation	Types of authorisation procedure can be the following: – Centralised (CP) – Mutual Recognition (MRP) – National (NP)
Date of Marketing Authorisation	Date in which the European Commission decision was released (Centralised Procedure) or date in which Regulatory Agency of Reference Member State granted the Marketing Authorisation (Mutual Recognition Procedure)
Marketing Authorisation Holder (MAH)	Company holding Marketing Authorisation
Orphan status	If the medicinal product is intended for the diagnosis, prevention or treatment of a life-threatening or chronically debilitating condition affecting less than 5 per 10.000 persons in the community and/or that without incentives it is unlikely that the marketing would generate sufficient return to justify the necessary investment (Reg. EC/141/2000)

Table 2
Disease classification

Paediatric therapeutic interest	The paediatric therapeutic interest of the medicinal product is 1. drugs included in the lists of Therapeutic Needs; 2. drugs included in the priority lists; 3. drugs included in the orphan drugs lists; 4. none.
Therapeutic area	Disease treated by the product

Table 3
Therapeutic indication

Approved indication	The granted indication for the Marketing Authorisation resulting from the assessment of the quality, safety and efficacy data submitted by MAH.
Lowest approved age/population	The lowest age for which the medicinal product has been approved.
Relevant adverse reactions	Any relevant adverse reaction.
Information on how to prescribe	How to dispense the medicinal product: without prescription (over the counter), repeat prescription, etc.

or social status. The proper use of medicines is dependent upon a wide dissemination of relevant information to all interested stakeholders (Regulatory Agencies, medical doctors, pharmacists, patient associations, industries, etc.).

Table 4
Developmental status

Existing paediatric studies	List of completed studies that recruited also children, with the following information: Type of study Description of the study aim (e.g. efficacy, safety, dose-finding). Sample size The number of patients enrolled in the study. Randomisation Study participants are assigned to groups in such a way that each participant has an equal chance of being assigned to each treatment (or control) group. Blinding The process through which one or more parties to a clinical trial are unaware of the treatment assignments. In a single-blinded study, the subjects are unaware of the treatment assignments. In a double-blinded study, both the subjects and the investigators are unaware of the treatment assignments. Controlled study A comparison group of study subjects who are not treated with the investigational agent. Type of control The subjects in the group may receive: 1. no therapy, 2. a different therapy (competitor), 3. a placebo. Age population Specifying the age of children recruited in the study.
Other known use in paediatrics	Any use of the active substance considered off-label.

Table 5
Medicinal product information

Availability in EU	List of EU countries where the medicinal product is available.
Formulation	List of all formulations (e.g. tablets, syrups) available divided by Country.
Packages	List of all the packages (e.g. package of 30 tablets/300 mg, ampoules) available divided by Country.
Price	Price to the public of the most used package for each Country.
Reimbursement regimen	Reimbursement regimen of the most used package for each Country.
Leaflet	PDF file of product leaflets.
Revision date	Product last revision date.

For many years, a lack of information on drugs continued to affect the paediatric population. It is well known that approved medicines are used in children without proper information on: dosage, potential toxicity, evidence of clinical safety and efficacy at the recommended dosages [1–3].

The specific issue of paediatric medicines has been considered by the European Institutions since 1997. For this purpose, a number of initiatives have been devel-

Table 6
Post-marketing modifications

Withdrawn medicinal product	Withdrawal of the Marketing Authorisation in the European Union.
Withdrawal date	Date of withdrawal of the product.
Reason for withdrawal	Detailed description of the reasons for the withdrawal.
Medicinal product safety announcement	Any recommended condition or restriction with regard to the safe and effective use of medicinal products.
Safety announcement motivation	Issues leading to the safety announcement.
Safety announcement date	Date of announcement.
Active substance safety announcement	Any recommended condition or restriction with regard to the safe and effective use of medicinal products.
Safety announcement motivation	Issues leading to the safety announcement.
Safety announcement date	Date of announcement.

oped within the last years, culminating with the entering into force of the European Paediatric Regulation [6] in January 2007.

The aim of this report is to present the status of paediatric medicines licensed by EMEA in the first 12 years of activity.

In details, we evaluated the number and the characteristics of medicines licensed for use in children by EMEA in the period October 1995 – December 2007.

Our analysis focused on new and innovative medicines authorised by EMEA, including the 'orphan drugs' subset, as defined by the Orphan Regulation n. 141/2000/EC [5].

4. Methodology

We examined the paediatric medicines registered in Europe under the EMEA Centralised Procedure (EMEA-CP) in the October 1995 – December 2007 period, deriving information stored in the European Paediatric Medicines Database (EPMD).

4.1. Data evaluated

The following parameters were assessed:

- Year of approval
- Active substance
- Anatomical Therapeutic Chemical – ATC code (first-level)
- Orphan Status
- Indication
- Age for which the drug is intended
- Paediatric Dosages

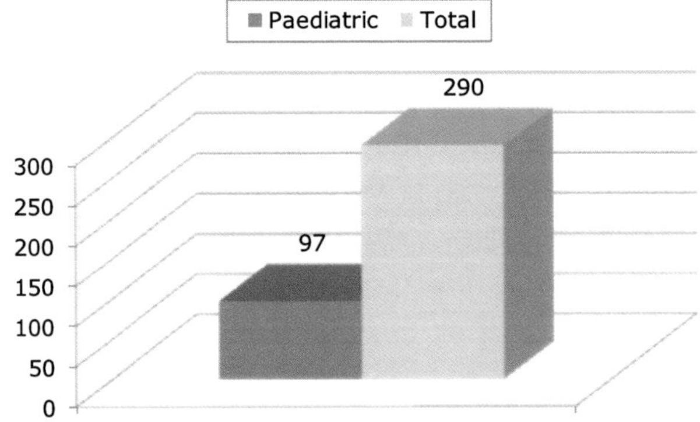

Fig. 1. Active substances authorised by EMEA (Oct. 1995 – Dec. 2007).

4.2. Analysis

Descriptive statistics were performed in order to identify the paediatric medicines approved by: a) year of Marketing Authorisation (MA), b) age of population for which the drug is approved, c) ATC code, and d) orphan status.

4.3. Definitions

- Paediatric medicines: medicines with registered labels including information to allow paediatric use. The inclusion of information about both label and Package Leaflet (PL) were related to paediatric indication and dosage (by age(s) and/or by weight).
- Paediatrics age groups: the groups of ages defined according to the ICH Topic E11 'Clinical Investigation of Medicinal Products in the Paediatric Population' Guideline (2000) [8].
- 'Orphan drugs' and 'Orphan-like drugs': as defined in the Regulation n. 141/2000/EC [5] and in the "Status Report on the implementation of the European Parliament Legislation on Orphan Medicinal Products" [4], respectively.

5. Results

5.1. General aspects

In the period October 1995 – December 2007, 290 active substances (AS) have been approved by EMEA under the Centralised Procedure, of which 97 include in their documentation (Summary of Product Characteristics – SPC/PL), information allowing paediatric use (Fig. 1).

Table 7
EMEA Paediatric and Orphan Medicines by ATC code

	Paediatric/Total		Orphan/Paediatric	
	N	%	N	%
J – Anti-infectives for systemic use	33/53	62	0/33	–
A – Alimentary tract and metabolism	18/34	53	10/18	55
L – Antineoplastic and immunomodulating agents	12/60	20	8/12	67
B – Blood and blood forming organs	9/22	41	0/9	–
R – Respiratory system	4/4	100	0/4	–
C – Cardiovascular system	2/15	13	2/2	100
D – Dermatologicals	3/4	75	0/3	–
S – Sensory organs	2/9	22	0/2	–
H – Systemic hormonal preparations, excluding sex hormones and insulins	3/10	30	1/3	33
N – Nervous system	4/26	15	2/4	50
V – Various	5/20	25	1/5	20
ALL other ATC	2/33	6	0/2	–
TOTAL	97/290	33%	24/97	25%

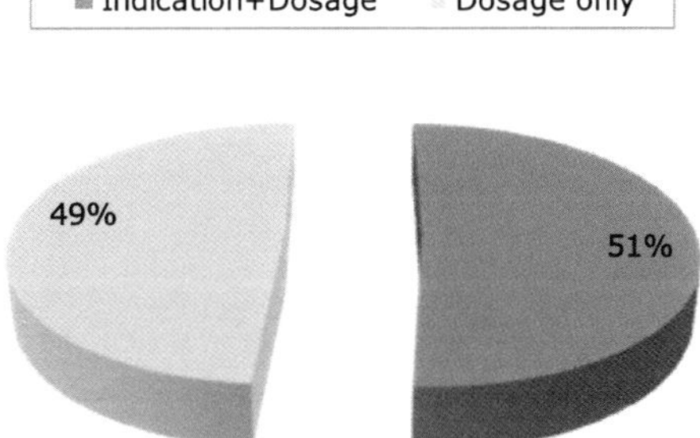

Fig. 2. Paediatric medicines authorised by EMEA (Oct. 1995 – Dec. 2007).

In particular, out of the 97 paediatric medicines, 51% were granted both a paediatric indication and dosage, and 49% included a paediatric dosage only (Fig. 2).

The ages reported in the MA documentation are of a wide range and only rarely correspond to the 5 age categories as stated in the ICH/E11. Moreover, the number of medicines approved for younger children is lower than those for older ones (the percentage being 9.4% and 23.4% in the newborn and in the infant groups, respectively).

5.2. ATC and orphan status

Authorised paediatric medicines belong to 11 ATC first-level categories. The percentage of paediatric medicines for each therapeutic area significantly varies among ATC codes: J-ATC (anti-infectives for systemic use) represents the group with the highest ratio, while C-ATC (Cardiovascular system) and S-ATC (Sensory organs) the lowest ones. Table 7 provides additional details.

Table 8
Paediatric orphan drugs and ATC distribution

ATC	Orphan drugs authorised	Paediatric orphan drugs authorised	Percentage
A	11	10	90.9
B	1	0	–
C		2	66.6
G	1	0	–
H	2	1	50
L	18	8	44.4
N	4	2	50
V	2	1	50
Not assigned yet	1	0	–
TOTAL	43	24	56%

Referring to orphan drugs, in the period October 1995 – December 2007, out of the 43 orphan drugs authorised by the EMEA, 24 were paediatric orphan drugs (Table 8).

Comparing the rate of paediatric medicines in orphan and non-orphan drug groups, a significant difference in favour of paediatric medicines in the orphan drug group is still noted (56% and 33%, respectively).

5.3. Discussion and conclusions

The results of the present study show that 33% of all medicinal products approved by EMEA are intended for the paediatric population, and that this percentage has remained more or less constant in the 12 years of activity of the Agency.

Moreover, the age for which the drug is indicated is still not compliant with the 5 age categories listed in the ICH/E-11 [8], varying case by case and potentially leading to both an increase in therapeutic errors and an actual difficulty in correctly prescribing drugs and avoiding possible 'off-label' use [7,9,10].

Notwithstanding this disappointing situation, a positive trend can be observed in the approval of paediatric medicines referred to some therapeutic areas of great paediatric interest (i.e. neurology, cardiovascular). In particular, if we consider orphan diseases, out of 43 authorised orphan drugs, 56% were specifically authorised for use in children.

In conclusion, since the implementation of the Centralised Procedure, a positive trend in the approval of safe and efficacious medicines for children seems to be in progress in Europe.

This trend is expected to increase rapidly in the future as a result of the adoption of the Paediatric Regulation, aimed at increasing the Europe-wide availability of high quality medicines specifically tailored to children.

Nevertheless, it is essential that information on medicinal products for paediatric use are made publicly accessible and data should be verified and controllable. The EMEA has recently made public many information on medicines authorised in EU through the EudraPharm database (http://eudrapharm.eu/eudrapharm/).

In addition to EudraPharm, TEDDY EPMD grants access to the main information related to paediatric medicines, some of which are not available in any other database. We deem this aspect a useful service to end users and a valid support to Regulatory Authorities.

Acknowledgements

This report is part of the Task-force in Europe for Drug Development for the Young (TEDDY) Network of Excellence supported by the European Commission's Sixth Framework Program (Contract n. 0005216 LSHBCT- 2005-005126).

References

[1] A. Ceci, M. Felisi, P. Baiardi, F. Bonifazi, M. Catapano, C. Giaquinto, A. Nicolosi, M. Sturkenboom, A. Neubert and I. Wong, Medicines for children licensed by the European Medicines Agency (EMEA): the balance after 10 years, *Eur J Clin Pharmacol* **62**(11) (2006 Nov), 947 952,Epub 2006 Oct 5.

[2] A. Ceci, M. Felisi, M. Catapano, P. Baiardi, L. Cipollina, S. Ravera, S. Bagnulo, S. Reggio and G. Rondini, Medicines for children licensed by the European Agency for the Evaluation of Medicinal Products, *Eur J Clin Pharmacol* **58**(8) (2002), 495–500

[3] European Commission Enterprise Directorate General, Better Medicines for Children. Proposed regulatory actions on paediatric medicinal products, *Eudralex* (2002).

[4] European Medicines Agency (EMEA), Status Report on the implementation of the European Parliament Legislation on Orphan Medicinal Products, **EMEA/7381/01** (March 30th 2001).

[5] European Parliament and Council Regulation 141/2000/EC, 16 December 1999 on Orphan Medicinal Products, *Official Journal of the European Communities* **L018/1** (22.01.2000).

[6] European Parliament and Council Regulation (EC) No 1901/2006, 12 December 2006, on medicinal products for paediatric use and amending Regulation (EEC) No 1768/92, Directive 2001/20/EC, Directive 2001/83/EC and Regulation (EC) No 726/2004. *Official Journal of the European Union* **L378** (12.12.2006), 1 19.

[7] M.A. Ghaleb, N. Barber, B.D. Franklin and I.C.K. Wong, What constitutes a prescribing error in paediatrics? *Qual Saf Health Care* **14** (2005), 352–357

[8] ICH Clinical Investigation of Medicinal Products in the Paediatric Population, ICH/Topic E11, *Eudralex* (2000).

[9] G. Koren, Z. Barzilay and M. Greenwald, Tenfold errors in administration of drugs doses: a neglected iatrogenic diseases in paediatrics, *Paediatrics* **77** (1986), 848–849.

[10] G.W. 't Jong, P.D. van der Linden, E.M. Bakker, N. van der Lely, I.A. Eland, B.H. Stricker and J.N. van den Anker, Unlicensed and off-label drug use in a paediatric ward of a general hospital in the Netherlands, *Eur J Clin Pharmacol* **58**(4) (2002), 293–297.

Pharmaceuticals Policy and Law 11 (2009) 41–49
DOI 10.3233/PPL-2009-0209
IOS Press

Off-label and unlicensed use of medicines for children

A. Neubert[a], M. Felisi[b], A. Bonifazi[b], C. Manfredi[b], I.C.K. Wong[a] and A. Ceci[b,*]
[a]*Centre for Paediatric Pharmacy Research, The School of Pharmacy and Institute of Child Health, University of London, London, UK*
[b]*Consorzio per Valutazioni Biologiche e Farmacologiche, Pavia, Italy*

The lack of specific drugs and labelling recommendations for the paediatric population is a long-standing problem.
Physicians frequently prescribe marketed medicines as off-label on the basis of clinical practice and medical knowledge. Moreover 'unapproved' drugs are employed in different formulations, routes, combinations to adapt them to children.
TEDDY studied the definitions of off-label and unlicensed use of medicines in paediatrics as defined by regulatory agencies and by scientific literature. This study confirmed the need for a common definition for unlicensed and off-label uses to be incorporated into the European legislation.
On the basis of the results of this investigation, TEDDY conducted a survey in order to reach a common definition with the intention to favour the use of a European official regulatory terminology and facilitate pharmaco-epidemiological research.
The definitions will be circulated within the scientific community and recommended to be adopted by relevant regulatory authorities.

Keywords: TEDDY, off-label, unlicensed, paediatric medicine, definition

1. Introduction

The lack of specific drugs and labelling recommendations for the paediatric population is a long-standing problem.

Physicians frequently prescribe marketed medicines as off-label on the basis of clinical practice and medical knowledge. Moreover 'unapproved' drugs are employed in different formulations, routes, combinations to adapt them to children.

Even if the use of 'off-label' and 'unlicensed' drugs in children is wide spread in Europe and worldwide, there is no common scientific and regulatory approach to this phenomenon and, in particular, a shared definition is missing. In Europe, this circumstance is still hindering the collection of reliable pharmaco-epidemiological data on a standardised basis.

TEDDY studied the definitions of off-label and unlicensed use of medicines in paediatrics as defined by regulatory agencies and by scientific literature. On the

*Corresponding author: Adriana Ceci, Consorzio per Valutazioni Biologiche e Farmacologiche, Via Palestro 26, 27100 Pavia, Italy. Tel.: +39 0382 25075; Fax: +39 0382 536544; E-mail: aceci@ cvbf.net.

basis of the results of this investigation, TEDDY designed and conducted a survey in order to reach a common definition with the intention to favour the use of a European official regulatory terminology and facilitate pharmaco-epidemiological research.

2. Regulatory definitions

2.1. US definitions

The Off-Label use has been firstly defined according to the Food and Drug Administration (FDA) rules as an 'unapproved use of a licensed drug' or as an use 'outside the terms of the licensed label'. In the latter definition Licensed Label stands for 'the official description of a drug product', which includes:

1) indication (what the drug is used for);
2) who should take it;
3) adverse events (side effects);
4) instructions for uses in pregnant women, children, and other populations and
5) safety information for patients.

In the FDA Modernization Act [16], the off-label use has been defined as: 'The use for indication, dosage form, dose regimen, population or other use parameter not mentioned in the approved labelling'.

2.2. EU definitions

In the European Union the Label (labelling) is defined according to Directive 2001/83/EC on the Community code relating to medicinal products for human use (art.1) [14] as the 'information on the immediate or outer packaging' while the 'Package leaflet' is 'a leaflet containing information for the user which accompanies the medicinal product'.

The product license corresponds to the Marketing Authorisation and an 'unlicensed product' should be better defined as 'unauthorised product'.

In October 2004, a document focusing on Adverse Events and off-label use in children has been released by EMEA. In this document [12], the terms 'off-label' and 'unlicensed' are included but not defined.

Moreover, no definition can be found in any other relevant EU documents or guidelines [13].

Finally, a definition of 'off label' use is not included in the new EU Regulation on medicinal products for paediatric use [15] that aims at avoiding the administration of 'medicines not authorised for use in children'. However, in its 'Better Medicines for children' document [11], the European Commission speaks about off-label as the 'use of product authorised for adults – products that have not been tested or authorised for paediatric use'. The same document refers also to the use of 'completely unauthorised products with the associated risks of inefficacy and/or adverse reactions (side effects)'.

Table 1
Definitions of off-label use

Definition	Reference No.
Off-Label is considered as the use of a marketed drug outside of the term of the product license or the Marketing Authorisation (MA) with reference to:	1–10, 17, 19, 21, 23–25, 27–29
Indication	1, 4, 5 6, 9, 10, 17, 23, 25, 27, 28, 29
Dose	1, 3, 4, 5, 6, 8, 9, 10, 17, 21, 23, 25, 27, 28 19, 29
Age	1, 3, 4, 5, 6, 8, 9, 10, 17, 19, 21, 23, 25, 27, 28, 29
Route	1, 3, 4, 5, 6, 8, 9, 10, 17, 21, 23, 25, 27, 28, 29
Contraindication	6, 8, 23, 27, 29
Formulation	4, 10, 19, 25

3. Literature review

An extensive literature review was carried out on the basis of the authors' previous knowledge, complemented by a systematic Medline search of documents published from 1995 through 2005 and containing the following combination of words: "child, drug, prescription, paediatric formulation, paediatric dosages, unlicensed, off-label". The literature search revealed a total of 66 publications relating to off-label or unlicensed drug use in children.

After a screening phase that revealed that 19 out of the 66 publications provided definitions for both off-label and unlicensed drug use [1–10,17,19,21,23–25,27–29], the most relevant papers providing useful definitions were further investigated and similarities and differences among the sources were evaluated.

Tables 1 and 2 list the commonest definitions respectively of off-label and unlicensed use found in literature.

These definitions have many similarities and some crucial differences. For instance, a different route of administration is considered both as 'off-label' [3,4,19] and as 'unlicensed' use [27,28].

The main differences encountered are shown in Table 3. They mainly revolve around the following issues:

a) Is the 'use of a drug outside the terms of the existing license' to be considered 'off-label' or 'unlicensed' with reference to the use that has been done?
b) Is the use of a drug in a form that requires a specific new marketing authorisation (like new formulation, new route of administration, new concentration, etc.) to be considered 'off-label' (being a modality of use not included in the MA documents) or 'unlicensed' (a new route is a 'type I or type II' variation for which a new authorisation is requested)?

Table 2
Definitions of unlicensed use

Definition	Reference No.
Unlicensed is considered as the use of a drug in lack of a product license or a MA for this use: Reasons considered for Unlicensed definition are:	1–10, 17, 19, 21, 23–25, 27–29
Modification to a licensed medicine (e.g. extemporaneous preparation)	4, 5, 6, 8, 9, 17, 21, 23, 25, 27, 28, 29
Particular formulation manufactured under a 'Special license'	4, 5, 6, 8, 23, 29
Chemicals and other substances used as medicines	8 6, 9, 23, 25, 29
Medicines used prior to the granting of a license (compassionate or experimental use)	4, 6, 8, 9, 23, 25, 29
Imported medicines	4, 6, 8, 9, 23, 25, 29
Contraindication	3, 27
Dosage not done in the Summary Product Characteristics or Patient Leaflet	3, 27
Different formulation	27
Different route	27

Table 3
Differences in the definition of off-label and unlicensed use

Condition	Off-label (Reference No.)	Unlicensed (Reference No.)
Dosage not done in the SPC or PL	4	27
	19	
	3	3
Contraindication	6	3
		27
Different route	4	27
	19	
	3	
Different formulation	4	27

c) Is the use of chemicals and other active substances aimed to prevent, make a diagnosis or cure human diseases (like chemicals, biological, nutritional, herbal, etc.) to be considered as an 'unlicensed' use of a medicinal product?
d) Is the use of experimental drugs after the end of the trials for which the drug has been authorised, an 'unlicensed' use?
e) Should an 'off-label' use, done with the purpose to investigate specific drug characteristics (dosage, effects, ADRs), be considered an 'experimental use' that requires a specific authorisation?

The effects of non-standardised definitions could hinder the development of well-standardised pharmaco-epidemiological surveys in different settings and European

UNLICENSED

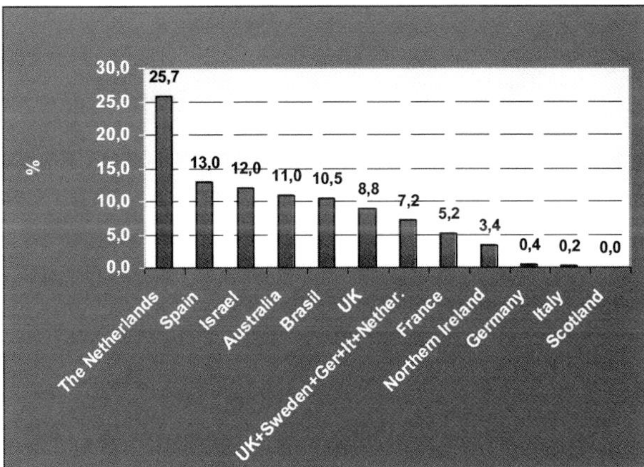

OFF-LABEL

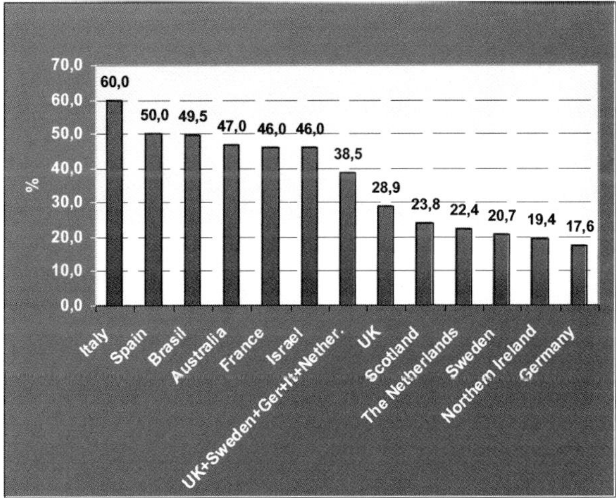

Fig. 1. Distribution of unlicensed and off-label use in different countries.

regions. Figures 1 and 2 show the incidence of 'off-label' and 'unlicensed' uses according to the papers surveyed. It cannot be excluded that the extreme variability observed (e.g. the case of Italy) also depends on the use of a different classification.

Moreover, efficacious regulatory actions could be prevented. In this perspective, it should be considered that the actions against off-label and unlicensed use ought to be different. For example, whereas off-label use is generally accepted by Health Authorities and not considered as a crime, the use of an unlicensed drug could expose health practitioners to a legal and professional risk. In particular, the FDA recognizes

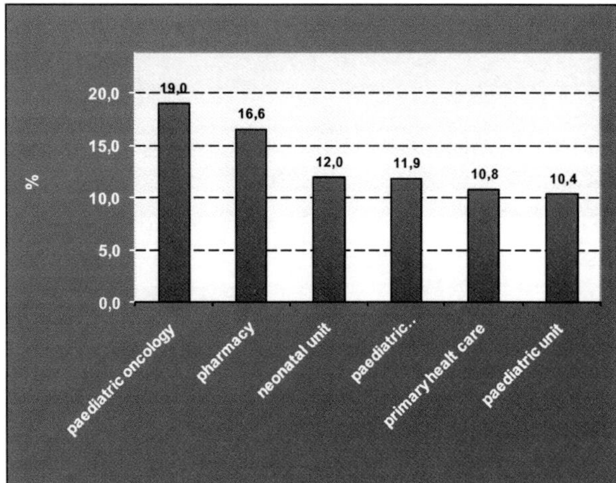

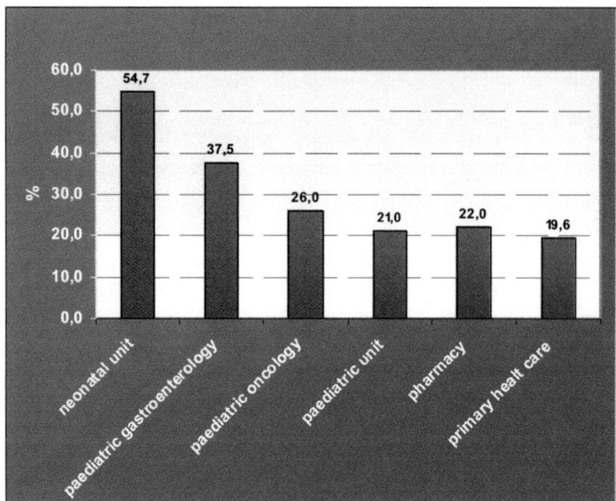

Fig. 2. Distribution of unlicensed and off-label use in different settings.

that 'off-label use of drugs by prescribing physicians is often appropriate and may receive endorsement from published literature', but at the same time the FDA policy is that 'Pharmaceutical Manufacturers cannot proactively discuss off-label uses, nor may they distribute written materials (promotional pieces, reprints of articles, etc.) that mention off-label uses' [30]. In Europe, an official off-label use policy has not been developed and unfortunately, the new Paediatric Regulation does not clarify this aspect [15].

4. Consensus definitions

The results of the literature review became the basis on which TEDDY designed and conducted a Delphi survey (questionnaire) using a web-based application [18, 20,22,26] to obtain consensus on common definitions for unlicensed and off-label use of medicines in children in order to favour the use of a European official regulatory terminology and facilitate pharmacoepidemiological research. Two on-line questionnaires were circulated iteratively among experts in the field in order to build the consensus by moving from concerns, scenarios and rules towards the following shared definitions:

"Off-label use" means 'all uses of a marketed drug not detailed in the SPC including therapeutic indication, use in age-subsets, appropriate strength (dosage), pharmaceutical form and route of administration.'

"Paediatric off-label use" specifically includes: 'all paediatric uses of a marketed drug not detailed in the SPC with particular reference to:

- therapeutic indication
- therapeutic indication for use in subsets
- appropriate strength (dosage by age)
- pharmaceutical form
- route of administration'

"Unlicensed use" means 'all uses of a drug which has never received a European Marketing Authorisation as medicinal for human use in either adults or children'.

5. Conclusions

This study confirmed the need for a common definition for unlicensed and off-label uses to be incorporated into the European legislation.

The need for a common definition is mainly derived from the fact that controversies on these definitions still exist in published contributions where a heterogeneity of the definitions applied is evident.

TEDDY survey has mainly resolved these controversies by agreeing that uses referred to 'marketed drugs', i.e. drugs which have marketing authorisation, are to be considered 'off-label' whereas those referred to 'unmarketed drugs', i.e. drugs without marketing authorisation, are to be considered 'unlicensed'. Moreover, for the first time, a definition is proposed for the 'unlicensed' and 'off-label' use of medicines specifically targeted for the paediatric population.

The definitions will be circulated within the scientific community and recommended to be adopted by relevant regulatory authorities.

Acknowledgements

This report is part of the Task-force in Europe for Drug Development for the Young (TEDDY) Network of Excellence supported by the European Commission's Sixth Framework Program (Contract n. 0005216 LSHBCT-2005-005126).

References

[1] S. Avenel, A. Bomkratz, G. Dassieu, J.C. Janaud and C. Danan, The incidence of prescriptions without marketing product license in a neonatal intensive care unit . *Arch Pediatr* **7**(2) (Feb 2000), 143–147.

[2] R. Bucheler, M. Schwab, K. Morike, B. Kalchthaler, H. Mohr, H. Schroder, P. Schwoerer and C.H. Gleiter, Off label prescribing to children in primary care in Germany: retrospective cohort study, *BMJ* **324**(7349) (1 Jun 2002), 1311–1312.

[3] P.R. Carvalho, C.G. Carvalho, P.T. Alievi, J. Martinbiancho and E.A. Trotta, Prescription of drugs not appropriate for children in a Pediatric Intensive Care Unit, *J Pediatr (Rio J)* **79**(5) (Sep–Oct 2003), 397–402.

[4] S. Conroy, I. Choonara, P. Impicciatore, A. Mohn, H. Arnell, A. Rane, C. Knoeppel, H. Seyberth, C. Pandolfini, M.P. Raffaelli, F. Rocchi, M. Bonati, G. Jong, M. de Hoog and J. van den Anker, Survey of unlicensed and off label drug use in paediatric wards in European countries. European Network for Drug Investigation in Children, *BMJ* **320**(7227) (8 Jan 2000), 79–82.

[5] S. Conroy, J. McIntyre and I. Choonara, Unlicensed and off label drug use in neonates, *Arch Dis Child Fetal Neonatal Ed* **80**(2) (Mar 1999), F142–144; discussion F144–145.

[6] S. Conroy, C. Newman and S. Gudka, Unlicensed and off label drug use in acute lymphoblastic leukaemia and other malignancies in children, *Ann Oncol* **14**(1) (Jan 2003), 42–47.

[7] S. Conroy and V. Peden, Unlicensed and off label analgesic use in paediatric pain management, *Paediatr Anaesth* **11**(4) (Jul 2001), 431–436.

[8] J.S. Craig, C.R. Henderson and F.A. Magee, The extent of unlicensed and off-label drug use in the paediatric ward of a district general hospital in Northern Ireland, *Ir Med J* **94**(8) (Sep 2001), 237–240.

[9] A. Dick, S. Keady, F. Mohamed, S. Brayley, M. Thomson, B.W. Lloyd, R. Heuschkel and N.A. Afzal, Use of unlicensed and off-label medications in paediatric gastroenterology with a review of the commonly used formularies in the UK, *Aliment Pharmacol Ther* **17**(4) (15 Feb 2003), 571–575.

[10] S. Ekins-Daukes, P.J. Helms, C.R. Simpson, M.W. Taylor and J.S. McLay, Off-label prescribing to children in primary care: retrospective observational study, *Eur J Clin Pharmacol* **60**(5) (Jul 2004), 349–353. Epub 2004 May 14.

[11] European Commission Enterprise Directorate General, Better Medicines for Children. Proposed regulatory actions on paediatric medicinal products. Consultation document, *Eudralex* (February 2002).

[12] European Medicines Agency (EMEA), Evidence of harm from off label or unlicensed medicines in children, *EMEA/11207/04* (26 Oct 2004).

[13] European Medicines Agency (EMEA), Guidelines on conduct of pharmacovigilance for medicines used by paediatric population, *EMEA/CHMP/PhVWP/235910/2005- rev.1* (25 January 2007).

[14] European Parliament and the Council of the European Union, Directive 2001/83/EC of the European Parliament and of the Council of 6 November 2001 on the Community code relating to medicinal products for human use, *Official Journal of the European Communities* **L 311** (28.11.2001), 67–128.

[15] European Parliament and Council Regulation (EC) No 1901/2006, 12 December 2006, on medicinal products for paediatric use and amending Regulation (EEC) No 1768/92, Directive 2001/20/EC, Directive 2001/83/EC and Regulation (EC) No 726/2004. *Official Journal of the European Union* **L378** (12.12.2006), 1–19.

[16] Food and Drug Administration, Modernization Act, (1997).

[17] V .Gavrilov, M. Lifshitz, J. Levy and R. Gorodischer, Unlicensed and off-label medication use in a general pediatrics ambulatory hospital unit in Israel, *Isr Med Assoc J* **2**(8) (Aug 2000), 595–597.
[18] F. Hasson, S. Keeney and H. McKenna, Research guidelines for the Delphi survey technique, *J Adv Nurs* **32**(4) (Oct 2000), 1008–1015.
[19] P.J. Helms, S. Ekins Daukes, M.W. Taylor, C.R. Simpson and J.S. McLay, Utility of routinely acquired primary care data for paediatric disease epidemiology and pharmacoepidemiology, *Br J Clin Pharmacol* **59**(6) (Jun 2005), 684–690.
[20] M.R. Lynn, E.L. Layman and S.P. Englebardt, Nursing administration research priorities. A national Delphi study, *J Nurs Adm* **28**(5) (May 1998), 7–11.
[21] J. McIntyre, S. Conroy, A. Avery, H. Corns and I. Choonara, Unlicensed and off label prescribing of drugs in general practice. *Arch Dis Child* **83**(6) (Dec 2000), 498–501.
[22] H.P. McKenna, The Delphi technique: a worthwhile research approach for nursing?, *J Adv Nurs* **19**(6) (Jun 1994), 1221–1225.
[23] A. Neubert, H. Dormann, J. Weiss, T. Egger, M. Criegee-Rieck, W. Rascher, K. Brune and B. Hinz, The impact of unlicensed and off-label drug use on adverse drug reactions in paediatric patients, *Drug Saf* **27**(13) (2004), 1059–1067.
[24] C.P. O'Donnell, R.J. Stone and C.J. Morley, Unlicensed and off-label drug use in an Australian neonatal intensive care unit, *Pediatrics* **110**(5) (Nov 2002), e52.
[25] C. Pandolfini, P. Impicciatore, D. Provasi, F. Rocchi, R. Campi and M. Bonati, Italian Paediatric Off-label Collaborative Group, Off-label use of drugs in Italy: a prospective, observational and multicentre study, *Acta Paediatr* **91**(3) (2002), 339–347.
[26] C. Powell, The Delphi technique: myths and realities, *J Adv Nurs* **41**(4) (Feb 2003), 376–382.
[27] G.W. 't Jong, P.D. van der Linden, E.M. Bakker, N. van der Lely, I.A. Eland, B.H. Stricker and J.N. van den Anker, Unlicensed and off-label drug use in a paediatric ward of a general hospital in the Netherlands, *Eur J Clin Pharmacol* **58**(4) (Jul 2002), 293–297. Epub 2002 Jun 15.
[28] G.W. 't Jong, A.G. Vulto, M. de Hoog, K.J. Schimmel, D. Tibboel and J.N. van den Anker, A survey of the use of off-label and unlicensed drugs in a Dutch children's hospital, *Pediatrics* **108**(5) (Nov 2001), 1089–1093.
[29] S. Turner, A. Longworth, A.J. Nunn and I. Choonara , Unlicensed and off label drug use in paediatric wards: prospective study, *BMJ* **316**(7128) (31 Jan 1998), 343–345.
[30] J. Woodcock, A shift in the regulatory approach, *Drug Information Association-Montreal (June 1997)*, http://www.fda.gov/cder/present/diamontreal/regappr/index.htm, accessed 23 September 2008.

Pharmaceuticals Policy and Law 11 (2009) 51–59
DOI 10.3233/PPL-2009-0210
IOS Press

Paediatric status and off-label use of drugs in children in Italy, United Kingdom and the Netherlands

M. Sturkenboom[a], M. Felisi[b], C. Manfredi[b], A. Neubert[c], L. Cantarutti[d], R. Padula[b], F. Sen[a] and K. Verhamme[a]

[a]*Pharmacoepidemiology Unit, Departments of Medical Informatics and Epidemiology & Biostatistics, Erasmus University Medical Center, Rotterdam, The Netherlands*

[b]*Consorzio per Valutazioni Biologiche e Farmacologiche, Pavia, Italy*

[c]*Centre for Paediatric Pharmacy Research, The School of Pharmacy and Institute of Child Health, University of London, London, UK*

[d]*Pedianet, Società Servizi Telematici, Padova, Italy*

Purpose. The differences in off-label prescriptions rate on the 5 most prescribed drugs in 14 ATC classes in 2005 were evaluated.

Methods. Prescription data on 143 drugs were extracted from 3 primary care research databases. Off-label was defined as the use of a drug below the Lowest Approved Age derived from the Summary of Products Characteristics.

Results. Only 25% of the drugs show the same Lowest Approved Age in all three Countries and 52% are currently used off-label in at least one (38%: UK, 40%: Holland, 46%: Italy). The percentage of off-label prescriptions varies from 4.7 (UK) and 7.6 (Italy) to 32.4 (The Netherlands).

Conclusions. Off-label prescriptions rate considerably varies in the three Countries due to the significant differences in the paediatric status. The Paediatric Regulation provides rules and incentives aimed at reducing the off-label uses in children. New criteria facilitating the paediatric status harmonisation should be urgently proposed.

Keywords: TEDDY, off-label, prescription, children

1. Introduction

The lack of drugs tailored for children is a long standing problem [1,7] and, as a consequence, drugs are used in newborns, infants, children and adolescents outside the terms of their Marketing Authorisations in relation to indication, dosage, age and route of administration both in Europe and worldwide [2–6,9,12,13,16]: these uses are regarded as "off-label". Many recent papers report that even if the 'off-label' use of drugs in children is wide spread in Europe and worldwide, significant differences in the extent of this use exist among Countries [11]. This is partially due to different cultures and current medical practices, but it is also explained by significant differences especially in the methodological approach used to assess and

*Corresponding author: Adriana Ceci, Consorzio per Valutazioni Biologiche e Farmacologiche, Via Palestro 26, 27100 Pavia, Italy. Tel.: +39 0382 25075; Fax: +39 0382 536544; E-mail: aceci@ cvbf.net.

profile off-label uses. To reduce variability in the data collection, information from well-standardised and homogenous prescription databases are needed.

Recently, TEDDY conducted a survey based on the Delphi methodology [10] to reach a consensus and propose a definition for the off-label use of medicinal products in children. The definition, which is also in compliance with the "paediatric status" definition provided in the Paediatric Regulation [8], could help in describing the use of drugs in the paediatric population in Europe with particular reference to the recognizable off-label uses.

The present study has been conducted within the TEDDY activities plan and aims at assessing the paediatric licensing status of drugs currently used in paediatric primary care and at comparing the extent of the off-label use in three European Countries: Italy, United Kingdom (UK) and The Netherlands.

2. Methods

2.1. Study sample

The study identified the 5 most frequently prescribed drugs per ATC Anatomic Level for each of the selected Countries and retrieved all data on the prescriptions of these drugs in 2005.

2.2. Sources of data

Information on the paediatric status were derived from the Summary of Product Characteristics (SPC), points 4.1 and 4.2, included in the National Formularies (*Prontuario Farmaceutico Nazionale – PNF* for Italy, *British National Formulary for Children- BNF-C* and the *Medicines Compendium* for the UK) or provided by National Agencies (*Medicines Evaluation Board – MEB* for The Netherlands).

Prescription data in children were extracted from 3 primary care research databases: the IMS Mediplus Disease Analyzer-Mediplus database (IMS-DA) in the UK [17], the PEDIANET database in Italy [14] and the Integrated Primary Care Information (IPCI) database [15] in The Netherlands. All 3 databases include the complete automated medical records of primary care physicians and exist in Countries where the primary care physician is the gatekeeper to health care.

Data stored in the databases include: active substance, medicinal product, Anatomical Therapeutic Chemical (ATC) category, age of patients, dosage, number of prescriptions per year.

2.3. Off-label status identification

According to the definition recently provided by TEDDY [10], 'off-label' is classified as all uses of a marketed drug that are not included in the SPC, with reference to indication, dosage, formulation, route of administration.

Table 1
The lowest age in the 3 countries

	United Kingdom		Italy		The Netherlands	
	N. of drugs	%	N. of drugs	%	N. of drugs	%
0–2 years	26	40.0	33	47.1	25	40.3
2–11 years	27	41.5	25	35.7	18	29.0
12–17 years	7	10.8	2	2.9	2	3.2
> 18 years	5	7.7	10	14.3	17	27.4
Total	65	100	70	100	62	100

For the purpose of this study, the following off-label uses were considered: a) use of a drug authorised only for adults (no paediatric indication reported in the SPC point 4.1); and b) use of a drug in patients younger than the approved age range given in the SPC (details on dosage by age as reported in the SPC point 4.2).

If the paediatric status for one active substance differed in various products, the lowest reported age was considered.

2.4. Data analysis

The number and percentage of off-label prescriptions were derived by crossing paediatric status and classes of ages for which the drug was prescribed. Frequencies of off-label prescriptions were stratified by drugs, drug categories (ATC) and classes of ages as reported in the databases (<2 years, 2–11 years and >11 years). Comparison across Countries was assessed by Chi-square test.

3. Results

The total number of mostly prescribed active substances in all ATC categories were 65 (UK), 70 (Italy) and 62 (The Netherlands), accounting to a total of 143 different drugs (in UK and Holland, less than 5 drugs were prescribed in the V, P and S ATC categories). Forty medicines were present in two databases contemporarily, while 14 in all three.

Drugs in the selected sample correspond to a total of 269590 prescriptions, of which 195021 were from UK, 52772 from Italy and 21797 from The Netherlands (77%, 68% and 62% of the total prescriptions in each database respectively).

3.1. Paediatric status

The paediatric status of the 143 drugs included in the study was derived from the minimum age given in the SPCs (Table 1). Results show a similar distribution among the age groups in Italy and UK, whereas in The Netherlands the percentage of prescription of drugs approved only for adults is higher (27.4%).

Moreover, only 8 of the drugs present in at least two databases have a similar approved minimum age (Table 2). Only 2 out of the 14 drugs present in all 3 databases have a common approved minimum age.

Table 2
Lowest age in the 40 drugs used in at least 2 Countries

ATC	Generic name	UK	Italy	The Netherlands
A03FA03	Domperidone	1 month	newborns	newborns
A06AD11	Lactulose	1 year	–	newborns
A07AA02	Nystatin	–	1 month	newborns
B02AA02	Tranexamic acid	children	children	–
B02BA01	Phytomenadione	newborns	newborns	newborns
C01CA24	Epinephrine	children	children	children
C03CA01	Furosemide	children	children	–
C05AA01	Hydrocortisone	–	12 years	no paediatric
C07AA05	Propranolol	newborns	–	children
C09AA02	Enalapril	children	–	children
D01AC01	Clotrimazole	children	no paediatric	–
D06AX01	Fusidic acid	newborns	–	no paediatric
D07AA02	Hydrocortisone	1 month	–	no paediatric
G03DC02	Norethisterone	no paediatric	–	no paediatric
H01BA02	Desmopressin	1 month	newborns	1 month
H02AB02	Dexamethasone	children	children	1 month
H02AB07	Prednisone	–	children	no paediatric
H03AA01	Levothyroxine sodium	1 month	newborns	newborns
J01CA04	Amoxicillin	–	newborns	newborns
J01CR02	Amoxicillin and enzyme inhibitor	–	2 months	newborns
J01FA09	Clarithromycin	–	6 months	newborns
J01FA10	Azithromycin	–	1 month	6 months
L01BA01	Methotrexate	children	newborns	children
L02AE04	Triptorelin	–	children	no paediatric
L04AA01	Ciclosporin	16 years	children	children
L04AX01	Azathioprine	children	–	children
M01AB05	Diclofenac	1 year	–	children
M01AE01	Ibuprofen	3 months	6 months	3 months
M01AE02	Naproxen	5 years	–	6 years
N02BE01	Paracetamol	2 months	newborns	3 months
N05BA01	Diazepam	1 year	newborns	children
N06BA04	Methylphenidate	6 years	–	6 years
P02CA01	Mebendazole	2 years	newborns	newborns
P03AC04	Permethrin	2 months	6 months	2 months
R03AC02	Salbutamol	children	1 month	newborns
R03BA01	Beclometasone	children	6 years	–
R06AE07	Cetirizine	2 years	1 year	–
S01AA13	Fusidic acid	all ages	–	no paediatric
S01GX04	Nedocromil	6 years	newborns	–
V03AC01	Deferoxamine	–	children	children

3.2. *Off-label uses by age categories*

Out of the 143 selected drugs, 75 (52%) are currently used in an unapproved age category (i.e. off-label) in at least one Country and, in particular: 25/65 (38%) drugs are used off-label in the United Kingdom, 25/62 (40%) in The Netherlands and 32/70 (46%) in Italy. Nine active substances are used off-label in the same age's population in at least 2 Countries while no drugs are simultaneously used off-label in all three

Table 3
Number of drugs used outside the approved age (off-label)

Drugs	Number	Percentage
In at last 1 country	75/143	52%
UK	25/65	38%
Italy	32/70	46%
The Netherlands	25/62	40%
In at least 2 country	9/40	22%
In all the 3 countries	0/14	0%

Countries (Table 3).

The distribution of off-label uses varies across the age groups and, as expected, a great number of drugs and prescriptions resulted off-label in children with less than 2 years-old in all the three Countries. Concerning the other classes of age (2–11 and 12–17 years), a high percentage of off-label use is observed in The Netherlands, while in the UK and Italy off-label prescriptions are negligible (Table 4).

3.3. Off-label uses by ATC categories

The percentage of off-label prescriptions is statistically different ($p < 0.001$) in the analysed Countries and varies from 4.7 (UK) and 7.6 (Italy) to 32.4% (The Netherlands) when all ATC categories are considered (Table 5).

A great variability is also shown across the different therapeutic categories. In particular, all drugs included in the *Cardiovascular System* category are used off-label in Italy, while in the UK very few prescriptions are reported off-label (41% vs 6%, $p<0.001$). In The Netherlands, 100% of the prescriptions in the *Genitourinary* category and 80% in the *Sensory Organ* and *Dermatology* groups resulted off-label, while in the other Countries the percentage of the off-label use appears to be significantly lower ($p < 0.001$).

4. Discussion

Our research demonstrates that 52% of the analysed drugs are used off-label in at least one Country; however, particularly in Italy and the UK, these drugs account for about 6% (4.7 and 7.6% respectively) of all issued prescriptions, while the majority of prescriptions are not off-label. This percentage is lower than the results published in a recent review conducted in Europe, Australia and USA, showing that the prevalence of off-label prescriptions in primary care varies from 11 to 37% [11]. On this basis, we can conclude that among primary care prescribers in the 3 Countries we have analysed, there is awareness regarding prescription liability and that this awareness is leading to a prudent prescription attitude in order to avoid any possible legal implication derived from off-label use.

Nonetheless, at the end of this discussion, a relevant unexpected result should also be considered. As described before, the Paediatric Status of drugs currently

Table 4
Off-label drugs and off-label prescriptions by age category

	United Kingdom			Italy			The Netherlands		
	Off-label / total drugs (%)	Off-label / total prescr.	% of prescr.	Off-label / total drugs (%)	Off-label / total prescr.	% of prescr.	Off-label / total drugs (%)	Off-label / total prescr.	% of prescr.
< 2 years	19/43 (44%)	7501/23036	33.0	27/57 (47%)	3381/16665	20.0	18/40 (45%)	1161/3618	32.1
2–11 years	10/62 (16%)	374/102659	0.4	11/68 (16%)	545/33155	1.6	19/61 (31%)	2984/11289	26.4
12–17 years	5/65 (8%)	1356/69326	2.0	6/61 (10%)	59/2952	2.0	16/57 (28%)	2925/6890	42.5
Total	25/65*	9231/195021	4.7	32/70*	3985/52772	7.6	27/62*	7070/21797	32.4

*Drugs could be used in more than 1 age group.

Table 5
Off-label drugs and off-label prescriptions by ATC category

	United Kingdom		Italy		The Netherlands	
	Off-label/ total prescription		Off-label/ total prescription		Off-label/ total prescription	
A – Alimentary tract and metabolism	202/6346	3%	0/2698	0%	20/1355	1%
B – Blood and blood forming organs	248/1048	23.70%	182/748	24.30%	13/178	7.30%
C – Cardiovascular system	99/1475	6.70%	48/117	41%	54/148	36.50%
D – Dermatologicals	828/27256	3%	825/2253	37%	3709/4662	80%
G – Genito-urinary system and sex hormones	1536/3976	38.6%	108/176	61.40%	1600/1600	100%
H – Systemic hormonal preparations, excluding sex hormones and insulins	19/1356	1.40%	23/4145	0.60%	104/289	36%
J – Anti-infectives for systemic use	345/41522	11%	0/2	9%	0/5435	68.80%
L – Antineoplastic and immunomodulating agents	17/154	0.10%	11/122	0.80%	nov-16	4.40%
M – Musculo-skeletal system	15/13551	0.10%	27/3533	0.80%	28/631	4.40%
N – Nervous system	0/20363	0%	apr-10	0.20%	8/748	1.10%
P – Antiparasitic products, insecticides and repellents	24/5105	0.50%	0/767	0%	2/171	1.20%
R – Respiratory system	1589/49871	3.20%	2199/13043	16.90%	154/4833	3.20%
S – Sensory organs	4309/22997	18.70%	547/2048	26.70%	1367/1729	79.10%
V – Various	0/1	0%	nov-17	64.70%	0/2	0%
Total	12244/195020	6.3%	3962/52772	7.5%	8517/22126	38.5%

used in children greatly differ in the three Countries even when the same active substance is concerned. As a consequence, the off-label prescriptions rate, still high in all Countries of the sample, varies considerably not only by age and therapeutic categories, but above all, by Country.

This result underlines that the differences in the Paediatric Status of the drugs used in paediatrics, instead of the different prescription habits or medical cultures as postulated by Pandolfini [11], represent the real reason of the variability reported by many European studies on the off-label use in children. We highlight that the Paediatric Status, assigned to a drug at the moment of a Marketing Authorisation (or a variation), is given on the basis of the proposal of the sponsor and after an assessment of the essential documentation submitted to an Institutional National or the European Regulatory Body. Data from our research demonstrate that a great variability exist among National Pharmaceutical Agencies in Europe in recognising the paediatric indication and dosages. These differences have to be clarified and it may be necessary to identify clear and reliable criteria to assign the paediatric status to the existing drugs. In lack of these criteria, drugs will continue to be considered in-label or off-label for different age groups in different Countries and any practical action to reduce such uses will be prevented.

The inventory of paediatric uses required by the Paediatric Regulation (Article 42) may represent the opportunity to compare the current use of drugs in different European Countries and to propose criteria for paediatric status harmonisation.

Acknowledgments

This study is part of the Network of Excellence TEDDY (Task-force in Europe for the Drug Development for the Young) supported by the EC Sixth Framework Program (Contract n. 0005216 LSHBCT-2005-005126).

References

[1] A. Ceci, M. Felisi, P. Baiardi, F. Bonifazi, M. Catapano, C. Giaquinto, A. Nicolosi, M. Sturkenboom, A. Neubert and I. Wong, Medicines for children licensed by the European Medicines Agency (EMEA): the balance after 10 years, *Eur J Clin Pharmacol* **62(11)** (2006), 947–952.

[2] I. Choonara and S. Conroy, Unlicensed and off-label drug use in children: implications for safety, *Drug Saf* **25** (2002), 1–5.

[3] C. Cowan, G. Hoskins and R.G. Neville, Clinical symptoms and 'off-label' prescribing in children with asthma, *Br J Gen Pract* **57**(536) (2007), 220–222.

[4] A. Cras, M.A. Conscience, G. Rajzbaum, A. Lillo-Le Louët, N. Lopez, I. Tersen and Y. Bezie, Off-label prescribing in a French hospital, *Pharm World Sci* **29**(2) (2007), 97–100. Epub 2006 Dec 12.

[5] M. Dell'Aera, A.R. Gasbarro, M. Padovano, N. Laforgia, D. Capodiferro, B. Solarino, R. Quaranta and A.S. Dell'Erba, Unlicensed and off-label use of medicines at a neonatology clinic in Italy, *Pharm World Sci* **29**(4) (2007), 361–367. Epub 2007 Mar 10

[6] E.R. Di Paolo, H. Stoetter, J. Cotting, P. Frey, M. Gehri, M. Beck-Popovic, J.F. Tolsa, S. Fanconi and A. Pannatier, Unlicensed and off-label drug use in a Swiss paediatric university hospital, *Swiss Med Wkly* **136**(13–14) (2006), 218–222.

[7] EMEA, The European paediatric initiative: History of the Paediatric Regulation, *EMEA/17967/04 Rev 1* (July 2007).

[8] European Parliament and Council Regulation (EC) No 1901/2006, 12 December 2006, on medicinal products for paediatric use and amending Regulation (EEC) No 1768/92, Directive 2001/20/EC, Directive 2001/83/EC and Regulation (EC) No 726/2004. *Official Journal of the European Union* **L378** (12.12.2006), 1–19.

[9] L. Hsien, A. Breddemann, A.K. Frobel, A. Heusch, K.G. Schmidt and S. Läer, Off-label drug use among hospitalised children: identifying areas with the highest need for research, *Pharm World Sci* **30**(5) (2008 Oct), 497–502. Epub 2008 Jan 26.

[10] A. Neubert, I.C.K. Wong, A. Bonifazi, M. Catapano, M. Felisi, P. Baiardi, C. Giaquinto, C.A.J. Knibbe, M.C.J.M. Sturkenboom, M.A. Ghaleb and A. Ceci, Defining Off-label and Unlicensed Use of Medicines for Children: Results of a Delphi survey, *Pharmacol Res* **58**(5–6) (2008 Nov–Dec), 316–322. Epub 2008 Sep 18.

[11] C. Pandolfini and M. Bonati, A literature review on off-label drug use in children, *Eur J Pediatr* **164**(9) (2005), 552–558. Epub 2005 May 24.

[12] S.S. Shah, M. Hall, D.M. Goodman, P. Feuer, V. Sharma, C. Fargason Jr, D. Hyman, K. Jenkins, M.L. White, F.H. Levy, J.E. Levin, D. Bertoch and A.D. Slonim, Off-label drug use in hospitalized children, *Arch Pediatr Adolesc Med* **161**(3) (2007), 282–290.

[13] D. Stewart, A. Rouf, A. Snaith, K. Elliott, P.J. Helms and J.S. McLay, Attitudes and experiences of community pharmacists towards paediatric off-label prescribing: a prospective survey, *Br J Clin Pharmacol* **64**(1) (2007), 90–95. Epub 2007 Feb 23.

[14] M. Sturkenboom, A. Nicolosi, L. Cantarutti, S. Mannino, G. Picelli, A. Scamarcia, C. Giaquinto; NSAIDs Paediatric Research Group, Incidence of mucocutaneous reactions in children treated with nilfumic acid, other nonsteroidal antiinflammatory drugs, or nonopioid analgesics, *Pediatrics* **116**(1) (2005), e26–33. Epub 2005 Jun 1.

[15] A.E. Vlug, J. van der Lei, B.M. Mosseveld, M.A. van Wijk, P.D. van der Linden, M.C. Sturkenboom and J.H. van Bemmel, Postmarketing surveillance based on electronic patient records: the IPCI project, *Methods Inf Med* **38** (1999), 339–344.

[16] I.C. Wong, N. Basra, V.W. Yeung and J. Cope, Supply problems of unlicensed and off-label medicines after discharge, *Arch Dis Child* **91**(8) (2006), 686–688.

[17] I. Wong and M. Murray, The potential of UK clinical databases in enhancing paediatric medication research, *Br J Clin Pharmacol* **59**(6) (2005), 750–755.

Pharmaceuticals Policy and Law 11 (2009) 61–70
DOI 10.3233/PPL-2009-0207
IOS Press

Recommendations for drug development for children

M. Catapano[a], C. Manfredi[a], P. Paolucci[b], H. Cross[c], K. Verhamme[d], M.J. Mellado Peña[e], I. Grosch-Wörner[f], C. Knibbe[g] and A. Ceci[a,*]

[a]*Consorzio per Valutazioni Biologiche e Farmacologiche, Pavia, Italy*
[b]*Department of Mother and Child, University of Modena and Reggio Emilia, Modena, Italy*
[c]*University College London, London, UK*
[d]*Pharmacoepidemiology Unit, Departments of Medical Informatics and Epidemiology & Biostatistics, Erasmus University Medical Center, Rotterdam, The Netherlands*
[e]*Department of Paediatrics, Hospital Carlos III, Madrid, Spain*
[f]*Charité Universitätsmedizin Berlin, Berlin, Germany*
[g]*Department of Clinical Pharmacology, San Antonio Hospital, Niewegein, The Netherlands*

One of TEDDY objectives is to "to identify unmet therapeutic needs for the development and use of medicinal products in male/female children" and it is compliant with the new provisions established by the Paediatric Regulation.

Thus TEDDY set up 12 Therapeutic Experts Groups (TEGs) to identify the needs in some therapeutic areas of paediatric interest.

Starting from the Assessment Documents released by EMEA-PEG and later on by EMEA-PDCO, a total of 14 therapeutic areas were analysed.

TEDDY experts have identified 442 products that need to be specifically developed for children by either extending the current authorised indication or developing new indications. Moreover, the study shows that a total of 1480 studies (i.e. PK, dosage, efficacy, safety or long term safety) should be conducted in order to develop more drugs for children.

In the light of these results, it is reasonable to question if all these studies are absolutely necessary and consequently if there are enough children to be enrolled in the trials for the same therapeutic area.

It is imperative to adopt a procedure of selecting which drugs need to be developed for each therapeutic area in order to avoid repetitive and unnecessary trials in children.

Keywords: TEDDY, children, drug development, therapeutic needs, priority lists

1. Introduction

The Paediatric Regulation [16], entered into force in January 2007, establishes several obligations and incentives to stimulate and increase the number of medicines devoted for children.

One of the main pillars of the Paediatric Regulation is represented by the setting up of an inventory of the therapeutic needs of the paediatric population, as established by the Paediatric Committee (PDCO) after consultation with the Commission, the Member States and interested parties. The inventory, to be regularly updated, will

*Corresponding author: Adriana Ceci, Consorzio per Valutazioni Biologiche e Farmacologiche, Via Palestro 26, 27100 Pavia, Italy. Tel.: +39 0382 25075; Fax: +39 0382 536544; E-mail: aceci@ cvbf.net.

Table 1
TEDDY Therapeutic Experts Groups (TEGs)

1	Haematology/oncology
2	Infectious diseases
3	Immunology
4	Rheumatology
5	Neurology-neuromuscular and psychiatric diseases
6	Gastroenterology
7	Respiratory
8	Cardiology
9	Nephrology
10	Diabetes
11	Pain
12	Formulation

identify the existing medicinal products used by the paediatric population and highlight the therapeutic needs and the priorities for research and development. In this way, companies should be able to easily identify opportunities for business development; the PDCO should be able to better judge the need for medicinal products and studies when assessing draft paediatric investigation plans, waivers and deferrals; and healthcare professionals and patients should have an information source available to support their decisions as to which medicinal products to choose.

In this framework, one of TEDDY objectives is to "to identify unmet therapeutic needs for the development and use of medicinal products in male/female children" and a specific Work Package (WP4 – Addressing key therapeutic questions in children) has been devoted to achieve this aim.

2. TEDDY therapeutic expert groups

Twelve Therapeutic Experts Groups (TEGs) (Table 1), formed by both internal and external experts and including different expertises (clinicians, clinical trial scientists, paediatric pharmacologists and clinical methodology researchers, etc.) were set up in order to achieve WP4 main objective: "to address questions concerning therapies in children with different chronic and acute diseases".

In setting up the groups, *multidisciplinarity* was taken into account and for this reason experts groups were composed by clinicians, trialists, paediatric pharmacologists, methodologists, pharmacists, statisticians, academics, researchers. In this perspective, each TEG leader worked in order to guarantee the presence of every area of expertise. Up to now, more than 100 experts have been involved in the work of the TEGs.

TEDDY TEGs also made use of the cooperation of National and European Scientific Societies (Table 2).

The groups concentrated their activities on systematically analysing, supporting and providing additional information to the EMEA Paediatric Working Party (PEG) and PDCO lists of therapeutic need assessment, and in particular:

Table 2
National and European Scientific Societies collaborating with TEDDY

SIOP Europe
European Paediatric Cardiology Association (AEPC)
European Society for Paediatric Endocrinology (ESPE)
European Society for Paediatric Infectious Diseases (ESPID)
European Respiratory Society (ERS)
Società Italiana per le Malattie Respiratorie Infantili (SIMRI)
European Society for Paediatric Gastroenterology, Hepatology and Nutrition (ESPGHAN)
Gastro-Intestinal Committee of the ESPGHAN
Società Italiana di Pediatria (SIP)

- giving opinion and possibly consensus (giving support) to the list of needs proposed by the PEG/PDCO;
- giving opinion on the type of paediatric clinical studies (as indicated by the PEG/PDCO) that should be performed;
- providing, on the basis of all available scientific evidence, additional proposals to complete or modify the list;
- increasing awareness on the assessments also through consultation with external experts.

Every issue related to the difficulties in R&D of paediatric medicines intended for a specific therapeutic indication (i.e. PK, safety, tolerability, efficacy, new formulation/different dosage, *etc.*) was highlighted.

TEDDY Experts have proceeded in identifying for each therapeutic area the existing products authorised for adult use and not for paediatric use or for other paediatric age categories.

2.1. Work methodology

The starting point of work for each TEG was the documents on therapeutic needs assessment released by the EMEA Paediatric Working Party and Paediatric Committee. The Experts Groups were asked to comment and also provide new suggestions on the documents released for consultation by the EMEA [1–15].

Moreover, for some therapeutic areas drugs available on the marketplace from Countries of the TEDDY Partners (Europe and Israel) were identified with particular reference to:

- drugs authorised under the Centralised Procedure and broken down for the above cited therapeutic areas (October 1995 – September 2005). For this group of drugs, representing the new and innovative medicines authorised by the EMEA, it is possible to collect a set of information easily available.
- drugs selected by PEG and PDCO and broken down for the above cited therapeutic areas. This group includes drugs authorised under National or Mutual Recognition Procedures.

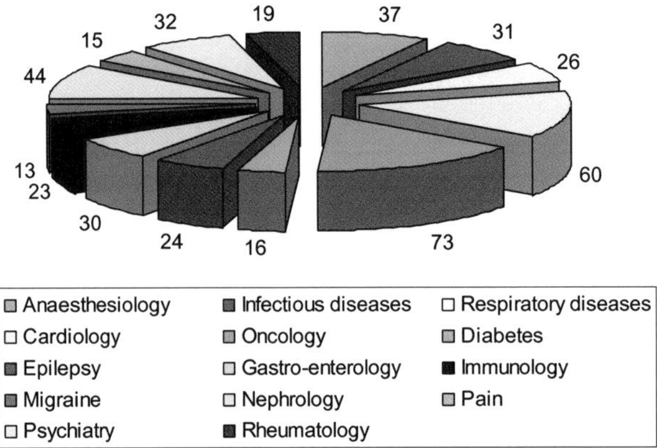

Fig. 1. Distribution of the selected products by therapeutic areas.

2.2. Experts evaluation

Expert groups of clinicians, clinical trial scientists, paediatric pharmacologists and clinical methodology researchers (TEDDY experts) were required to agree on a list of priority needs in key paediatric areas, and to make recommendations to Regulatory Agencies and sponsors.

In details, each experts group provided comments and suggestions on the docs above cited (EMEA PEG/PDCO Therapeutic Needs Assessment) in order to categorise and prioritise the therapeutic needs not covered by authorised treatment for children.

To better categorise the conditions/diseases treated by the examined drugs, the following classification was adopted:

- priority 0 = no interest for children since the drug is indicated for diseases which do not affect children;
- priority 1 = low priority for children since the drug is indicated for unserious diseases which affect both adults and children or diseases already cured in children;
- priority 2 = high priority for children since the drug is indicated for serious diseases which affect children and of which significant benefit compared with the existing methods could be derived by a new treatment.

3. Results

TEDDY experts have identified 443 products that need to be specifically developed for children in terms of extending the current authorised indication from adults to

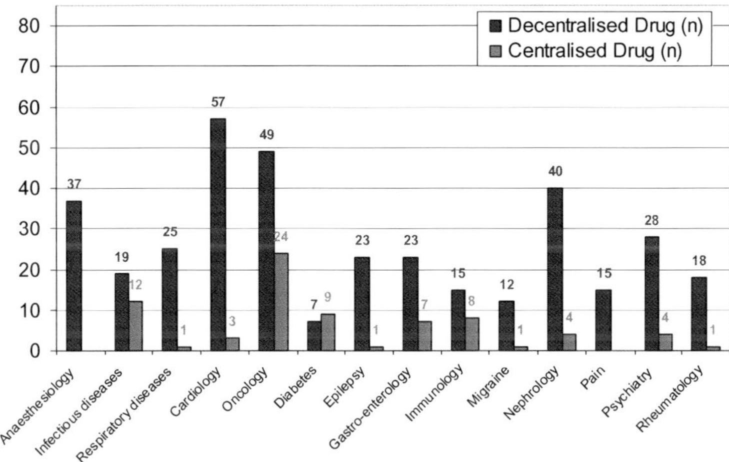

Fig. 2. Decentralised and Centralised products by therapeutic areas.

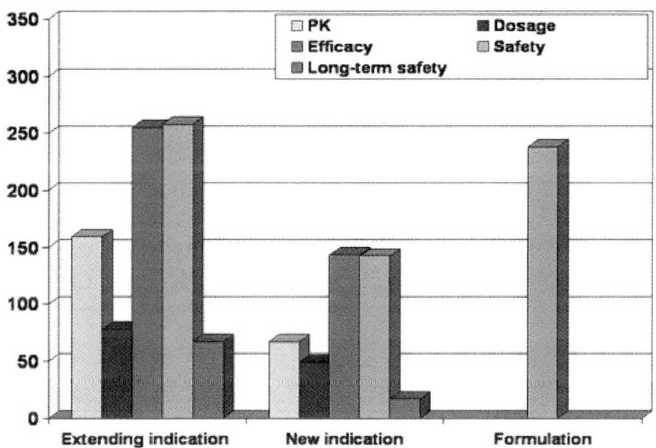

Fig. 3. Type of study requests by extending indication or new indication or formulation.

children or from older to younger children or in terms of developing new indications. A total of 14 therapeutic areas were analysed, as shown in Fig. 1.

On a total of 443 products, 75 were products authorised under the centralised procedure. The distribution of drugs both authorised under the Centralised and Decentralised (National and/or Mutual recognition) procedures is shown in Fig. 2.

A total of 1473 studies are requested in order to develop products of paediatric interest. The details of the type of studies requested (PK, dosage, efficacy, safety or long term safety) are shown in Fig. 3.

Tables 3 and 4 include details of the products by therapeutic areas, Table 5 includes details on requests related to age appropriate formulations.

Table 3
Requests of studies by therapeutic areas for developing new indications

Therapeutic classes	Drugs (n)	PK	Dose	Efficacy	Safety	Long-term safety
Anaesthesiology	2			1	1	
Infectious diseases	2	1		1	1	
Respiratory diseases	16	5	1	16	14	
Cardiology	7		7	7	7	
Oncology	32	25	8	29	29	
Diabetes	1	1		1	1	
Epilepsy	5		2	5	5	
Gastro-enterology	20	6	7	19	20	5
Immunology	14	4	6	11	11	
Migraine	2		2	2	2	
Nephrology	29	21	8	29	29	1
Pain	1			1	1	
Psychiatry	9	4		9	9	5
Rheumatology	12		8	12	12	6
Total	152	67	49	143	142	17

Table 4
Requests of studies by therapeutic areas for extending current authorised indications

Therapeutic classes	Drugs (n)	PK	Dose	Efficacy	Safety	Long-term safety
Anaesthesiology	26	12	4	12	14	4
Infectious diseases	28	24		27	27	2
Respiratory diseases	19	5	11	16	17	9
Cardiology	52	2	41	44	43	6
Oncology	44	26		35	35	1
Diabetes	16	12		15	15	4
Epilepsy	15	11	3	8	9	2
Gastro-enterology	18	12	1	16	16	2
Immunology	12	2	5	8	8	3
Migraine	11	10		10	10	10
Nephrology	26	16	7	25	26	4
Pain	15	9	1	12	12	4
Psychiatry	25	18	2	23	23	15
Rheumatology	4		3	4	3	1
Total	311	159	78	255	258	67

To better categorise the conditions/diseases treated by the examined drugs, experts provided a sort of classification, identifying the priority of research in a sample of drugs as shown in Figs 4 and 5, according to the need of developing new indications and extending the current authorisation to paediatric populations.

4. Conclusions

The work carried out by the TEDDY TEGs shows that many studies are currently requested to develop more drugs for children.

Table 5
Requests of studies by therapeutic areas for developing age appropriate formulations

Therapeutic classes	Drugs (n)
Anaesthesiology	21
Infectious diseases	15
Respiratory diseases	8
Cardiology	50
Oncology	18
Diabetes	4
Epilepsy	17
Gastro-enterology	21
Immunology	11
Migraine	7
Nephrology	30
Pain	7
Psychiatry	15
Rheumatology	14
Total	238

Priority of research: developing new indication

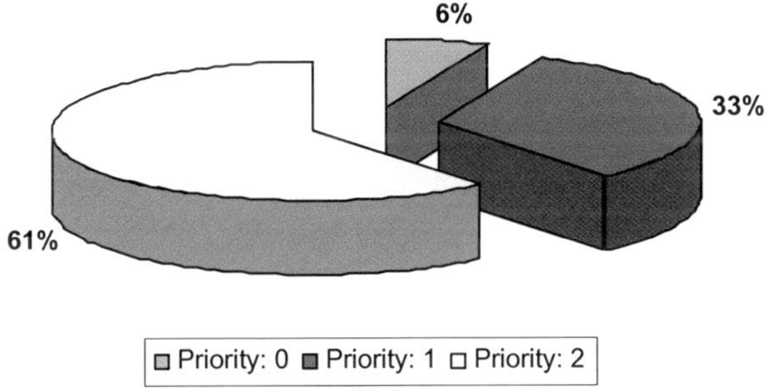

Legend: Priority 0 = no interest for children since the drug is indicated for diseases which do not affect children; Priority 1 = low priority for children since the drug is indicated for unserious diseases which affect both adults and children or diseases already cured in children; Priority 2 = high priority for children since the drug is indicated for serious diseases which affect children and of which significant benefit compared with the existing methods could be derived by a new treatment.

Fig. 4. Priority of research as defined by TEDDY experts (new indications) in a sample of 71 drugs.

More clinical trials will have a positive effects on the drug use rationale and on ADRs reduction in children. On the other hand, it is reasonable to question if all these studies are absolutely necessary and consequently, if there are enough children to be enrolled in the trials for the same therapeutic area.

Our study demonstrates that it is necessary to apply specific criteria to select

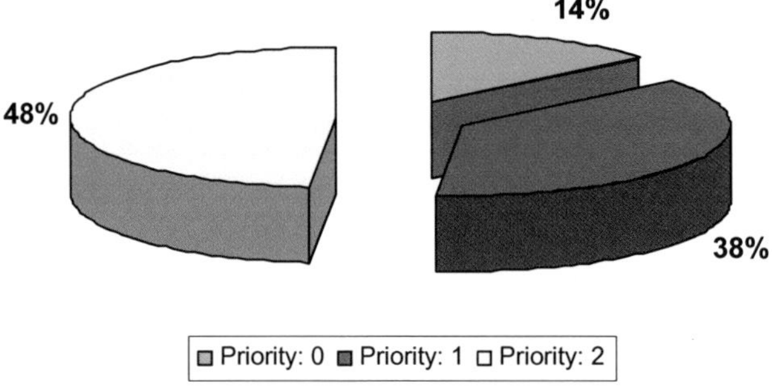

Legend: Priority 0 = no interest for children since the drug is indicated for diseases which do not affect children; Priority 1 = low priority for children since the drug is indicated for unserious diseases which affect both adults and children or diseases already cured in children; Priority 2 = high priority for children since the drug is indicated for serious diseases which affect children and of which significant benefit compared with the existing methods could be derived by a new treatment.

Fig. 5. Priority of research as defined by TEDDY experts (extending indications) in a sample of 148 drugs.

the medicinal products for which developmental efforts are absolutely needed and that through these criteria it will be possible to reduce the economic and research commitment by 6–14% (priority 1 and 2 studies only) up to 33–38% (priority 1 studies only).

A first reduction can be performed by selecting drugs belonging to the same therapeutic area and having the same level of interest of which only the more interesting should be proposed to be investigated and developed in children.

Moreover, integrating the results of this study with what emerged from the analysis carried out by TEDDY on the existing paediatric clinical trials (both registrative and non-registrative), we can demonstrate that good quality paediatric studies already exist for many active substances included in the therapeutic needs lists, thus they should not be repeated in vain. This also represents a criterion.

In conclusion, to define priorities TEDDY suggests the adoption of *at least* the following criteria:

- lack of any paediatric alternative treatments on the market;
- existence of therapeutic interest relevant for paediatrics;
- lack of evidences from paediatric clinical studies supporting the marketing authorisation of the currently available drugs used in children.

This selection criteria should be adopted not only by Pharmaceutical Companies, but also in European and National Research Programs in order to better concentrate public and private efforts on those drugs lacking of a specific indication for children and also of paediatric studies.

Acknowledgements

This report is part of the Task-force in Europe for Drug Development for the Young (TEDDY) Network of Excellence supported by the European Commission's Sixth Framework Program (Contract n. 0005216 LSHBCT-2005-005126).

We thank all experts for their invaluable contribution: Eugenio Baraldi, Hans Bisgaard, Gianni Bisogno, Attilio Boner, Andrew Bush, Carmen Cano, Modesto Carli, Silvia Carraro, Franco Chiarelli, Alfonso Delgado, Maria Esposito Salsano, Alberto Garaventa, J-M Gauthier, Moshe Gavish, Lut Goossens, Bertil Kagedal, Deirdre Kelly, Johan de Jongste, Peter Hindmarsh, Giuliana Lama, Svetlana Leschiner, Henrik Lövborg, María Jesús Mardomingo, Jean Paul Misson, Luigi Notarangelo, Curt Peterson, Roi Piñeiro, José Tomás Ramos, Riccardo Riccardi, Carmelo Rizzari, Pablo Rojo Conejo, Enriqueta Roman Riechman, Angelo Rosolen, Nicolino Ruperto, Annamaria Staiano, Ales Stuchlik, Dick Tibboel.

References

[1] European Medicines Agency (EMEA), Assessment of the paediatric needs – Pain, *EMEA/CHMP/189220/2005* (23 June 2005).
[2] European Medicines Agency (EMEA), Assessment of the paediatric needs – Rheumatology, *EMEA/CHMP/234105/2005* (18 July 2005).
[3] European Medicines Agency (EMEA), Assessment of the paediatric needs – Cardiovascular products, *EMEA/CHMP/327847/2005* (10 October 2005).
[4] European Medicines Agency (EMEA), Assessment of the paediatric needs - Chemotherapy products (Part I), *EMEA/CHMP/366844/2005* (15 November 2005).
[5] European Medicines Agency (EMEA), Assessment of the paediatric needs – Immunology, *EMEA/CHMP/405908/2005* (14 December 2005).
[6] European Medicines Agency (EMEA), Assessment of the paediatric needs – Epilepsy, *EMEA/377174/2006* (20 September 2006).
[7] European Medicines Agency (EMEA), Assessment of the paediatric needs – Diabetes type I and II, *EMEA/224688/2006* (02 June 2006).
[8] European Medicines Agency (EMEA), Assessment of the paediatric needs – Chemotherapy products (Part II) - Supportive therapy, *EMEA/224696/2006* (02 June 2006).
[9] European Medicines Agency (EMEA), Assessment of the paediatric needs – Migraine, *EMEA/224515/2006* (02 June 2006).
[10] European Medicines Agency (EMEA), Assessment of the paediatric needs – Anaesthesiology, *EMEA/405166/2006* (October 2006).
[11] European Medicines Agency (EMEA), Assessment of the paediatric needs – Antiinfectious therapy with focus on antimycotics, antivirals (except HIV), *EMEA/435350/2006* (October 2006).
[12] European Medicines Agency (EMEA), Assessment of the paediatric needs – Asthma and other obstructive chronic lung diseases EMEA/439727/2006(October 2006).
[13] European Medicines Agency (EMEA), Assessment of the paediatric needs – Nephrology, *EMEA/13306/2007* (December 2006).

[14] European Medicines Agency (EMEA), Assessment of the paediatric needs – Psychiatry, *EMEA/288917/2007* (27 July 2007).

[15] European Medicines Agency (EMEA), Assessment of the paediatric needs – Gastro-enterology, EMEA/527934/2007 (October 2007).

[16] European Parliament and Council Regulation (EC) No 1901/2006, 12 December 2006, on medicinal products for paediatric use and amending Regulation (EEC) No 1768/92, Directive 2001/20/EC, Directive 2001/83/EC and Regulation (EC) No 726/2004. Official Journal of the European Union L378 (12.12.2006), 1–19.

Pharmaceuticals Policy and Law 11 (2009) 71–78
DOI 10.3233/PPL-2009-0205
IOS Press

Clinical trials for paediatric medicines in Europe

P. Baiardi[a], S. Girotto[b], O. Della Pasqua[c], L. Harper[d], I. Grosch-Wörner[e], A. Ceci[a,*] and C. Giaquinto[b]
[a]*Consorzio per Valutazioni Biologiche e Farmacologiche, Pavia, Italy*
[b]*Azienda Ospedaliera di Padova, Padova, Italy*
[c]*Leiden/Amsterdam Center for Drug Research, Leiden, The Netherlands*
[d]*Medical Research Council, London, UK*
[e]*Charité Universitätsmedizin Berlin, Berlin, Germany*

For years the lack of studies specifically designed to investigate pharmacological and toxicological aspects in the paediatric population has forced children to use many approved drugs without a proper information on dosage, efficacy and safety and on the basis of data extrapolated from adults studies.

In Europe, the Directive EC/2001/20 on Good Clinical Practice, was the first to take into consideration the need of performing clinical trials in children in compliance with the current GCP requirements. Moreover, the Note for Guidance ICH Topic E11 gives recommendations on clinical trials' characteristics.

Our study found that under the EMEA centralised procedure, 60 drugs were licensed for use in children in the period 1995–2005. These data show an increasing trend in the percentage of EMEA approved medicines for children compared with previously reported figures.

Moreover, few clinical studies were performed in compliance with the paediatric age groups as defined by the ICH/E11 guideline. This is of particular concern especially when the adolescent age group is considered, since adolescents are frequently recruited together with adults.

The new Paediatric Regulation, in force from January 2007, is expected to dramatically change this situation.

Keywords: TEDDY, clinical trial methodology, paediatric medicines, Europe

1. Background

For years the lack of studies specifically designed to investigate pharmacological and toxicological aspects in the paediatric population has forced children to use many approved drugs without a proper information on dosage, efficacy and safety and on the basis of data extrapolated from adults studies in a more or less empiric way [1,2].

In Europe, the Directive EC/2001/20 on Good Clinical Practice (GCP) [3], entered into force in May 2004, was the first to take into consideration the need of performing clinical trials (CTs) in children in compliance with the current GCP requirements; in fact, it includes an ad hoc article (Article 4) that aims at guaranteeing that paediatric clinical research in Europe is conducted at the highest ethical level, using appropriate methodology, avoiding discomfort for children and after having obtained informed

*Corresponding author: Adriana Ceci, Consorzio per Valutazioni Biologiche e Farmacologiche, Via Palestro 26, 27100 Pavia, Italy. Tel.: +39 0382 25075; Fax: +39 0382 536544; E-mail: aceci@ cvbf.net.

consent from parents and assent from children, when applicable. Moreover, the Note for Guidance ICH Topic E11 [5] gives recommendations on CT characteristics, also specifying that paediatric patients should be given medicines that have been appropriately evaluated for their use, in all paediatric age groups. Particularly pharmacokinetic (PK) studies and short and long term safety evaluations are almost always required, and large efficacy trials, enrolling large paediatric populations, are needed only when extrapolation of results from adults is not recommended.

Notwithstanding these efforts, criticisms have been made, especially to the EC/2001/20 Directive that is blamed to double responsibility, bureaucracy and expenses. These circumstances seem to have prevented a wide Directive implementation and it is still a questionable matter whether or not these instruments have been included in clinical practice in order to change the attitude and the methodology to conduct paediatric CTs. As a consequence, a debate on the future of the EC/2001/20 Directive was opened at the European Commission level.

In order to contribute to this discussion, the aim of the present study is to evaluate the status of paediatric clinical trials performed for drugs to be used in children in order to verify their methodology and their compliance with the Note for Guidance ICH Topic E11 (ICH/E11).

2. Methods

2.1. Data source and sample

We evaluated medicines registered in Europe under the EMEA Centralised Procedure in the decade from October 1995 to September 2005 and whose label and package Leaflet (PL) include paediatric indication and/or dosage (by age(s) and/or by weight).

Paediatric age has been defined according to ICH/E11 guidelines and all drugs for children under 18 years were selected.

Data were derived from the TEDDY European Paediatric Medicine Database – EPMD (www.teddyoung.org).

2.2. Data collection and analysis

For each study evaluated, a number of variables were collected (Table 1). For the purpose of this analysis, data were entered in a database following a standard format based on a common terminology; validation checks were carried out to ensure integrity and consistency.

The scientific quality was guaranteed by a multidisciplinary team of experts.

Management and analysis were carried out using an Office Software Package.

All clinical trials (PD, PK, efficacy and safety) that were reported in the marketing authorization documentation (European Public Assessment Report – EPAR, available

Table 1
Data collected and stored in the database

GENERAL	ATC MEDICINAL PRODUCT ACTIVE SUBSTANCE DISEASE FORMULATION TYPE OF STUDY (PD/PK, EFFICACY, SAFETY)
PK STUDY	STUDY NUMBER ADULT PK (Y/N) DOSE (SINGLE/MULTIPLE/MISSING)) N° PARTICIPANTS AGE SEX
EFFICACY STUDY	STUDY NUMBER N° PARTICIPANTS AGE SEX COUNTRY (EUROPE, REST OF THE WORLD) MULTICENTRE BLINDING CONTROLLED (Y/N/MISSING) COMPARATOR (ACTIVE/PLACEBO) RANDOMIZATION (Y/N/MISSING) PRIMARY ENDPOINT DEFINED (Y/N)
SAFETY STUDY	STUDY NUMBER N° PARTICIPANTS AGE SEX COUNTRY (EUROPE, REST OF THE WORLD) MULTICENTRE BLINDING CONTROLLED (Y/N/MISSING) COMPARATOR (ACTIVE/PLACEBO) RANDOMIZATION (Y/N/MISSING) PRIMARY ENDPOINT DEFINED (Y/N)

at the EMEA website, www.emea.europa.eu) and had specific reference to paediatric age groups were studied in order to evaluate their compliance with ICH/E11 guideline (Table 2). To this end, paediatric medicines were categorised in 3 groups according to the disease which they are intended to treat and to the indications provided by the ICH/E11.

3. Results

Sixty drugs were granted a Marketing Authorisation (MA) for use in children in the decade 1995–2005 (Table 3).

A total of 188 paediatric clinical trials were included in their MA dossiers; in particular, of the 60 drugs, 58.3% included 1 to 3 paediatric trials, and 26.7% more

Table 2
Timing and type of paediatric development according to ICH/E11 guidance document

Disease	Timing of studies	Type of studies	
Predominantly or exclusively affecting paediatric patients (GROUP 1)	The entire development program will be conducted in children	PK, Efficacy Safety	
Serious or life-threatening conditions occurring in both adult and paediatric patients, with no or limited therapeutic options (GROUP 2)	Paediatric development should begin early, following phase 1 in adults and after potential benefit has been demonstrated	IF: Adult indications, similar disease process and outcomes	PK/(PD) in all the age ranges Safety
		IF: New indication, different course of the diseases or outcomes	PK in all age ranges Efficacy Safety
Other diseases or conditions (GROUP 3)	Limited paediatric data would be available at the time of the application, but more would be expected after Marketing Authorisation	Short and Long Term Safety	

than 3 studies. The majority of these CTs (87.4%) were conducted only in children. In the remaining, children were enrolled together with adults.

The characteristics of the analysed CTs are summarised below.

3.1. PK studies

A total of 77 PK studies in children were performed for 38 drugs (63%).

The total number of enrolled children was 1990.

PK data in the adult population were reported in all documentations and PK studies in the paediatric population were designed according to the results obtained in adults.

Only two studies took into account the age classification according to the ICH/E11 guideline (Pedea and Vfend), while the others considered different age groups and two drugs (Benefix and Xolair) performed studies in adults also including adolescents.

Ten studies included a classification of participants by gender, but no results by sex were reported.

3.2. Efficacy studies

A total of 135 efficacy studies (enrolling 11959 children) were included in the MA dossiers of 47 drugs.

Three drugs enrolled children together with adults (Xolair, Opatanol, Ferriprox), while other 4 performed both paediatric trials and adults trials recruiting also children (Refacto, Benefix, Advate, Aerius).

Table 3
List of analyzed drugs

ATC	Active substance	Medicinal product
J – Anti-infectives for systemic use	abacavir	Ziagen
	abacavir/lamivudine	Kivexa
	amprenavir	Agenerase
	efavirenz	Stocrin/Sustiva
	emtricitabine	Emtriva
	enfuvirtide	Fuzeon
	indinavir sulphate	Crixivan
	lamivudine	Epivir/Zeffix
	lamivudine/zidovudine	Combivir
	lopinavir/ritonavir	Kaletra
	nelfinavir	Viracept
	nevirapine	Viramune
	oseltamivir	Tamiflu
	palivizumab	Synagis
	ribavirin	Contronak/Rebetol
	ritonavir	Norvir
	stavudine	Zerit
	telithromycin	Ketek/Levviax
	variconazole	Vfend
A – Alimentary tract and metabolism	carglumic acid	Carbaglu
	imiglucerase	Cerezyme
	insulin and isophane (NPH)	Actraphane/Actrarapid/Mixtrad
	insulin, rDNA	
	insulin aspart	Novomix 30/Novorapid
	insulin determir	Levemir
	insulin glargine	Lantus/Optisulin
	insulin lispro	Humalog/Liprolog
	insulin rDNA	Monotard/Ultratard/Velosulin
	laronidase	Aldurazime
	mercaptamine bitartrate	Cystagon
	nitisinone	Orfadin
	phenylbutyrate	Ammonaps
	repaglinide	Novornorm/Prandin
	zinc acetate dihydrate	Wilzin
L – Antineoplastic and immunomodulating agents	aresenic trioxide	Trisenox
	basiliximab	Simulect
	daclizumab	Zenapax
	etanercept	Enbrel
	imatinib mesilate	Glivec
	interferon alfa-2b	Intron A/Viraferon
	mitotane	Lysodren
	mycophenolate mofetil	Cellcept
	temozolomide	Temodal
B – Blood and blood forming organs	darbepoetin alfa	Aranesp/Nespo
	epoetin beta	Neorecormon
	human C protein	Ceprotin
	human coagulation factor IX	Nonafact

Table 3, continued

ATC	Active substance	Medicinal product
	moroctocog alfa	Refacto
	nonacog alfa	Benefix
	octocog alfa	Advate/Helixate Nexgen/Kogenate Bayer
R – Respiratory system	desloratadine	Aerius/Allex/Azomyr/Neoclarityn/Opulis
	nitric oxide	Inomax
	omalizumab	Xolair
C – Cardiovascular system	bosentan	Tracleer
	ibuprofen	Pedea
D – Dermatologicals	eflornitine	Vaniqa
	tacrolimus	Protopic/Protopy
S – Sensory organs	emedastine difumarate	Emadine
	olopatadine	Opatanol
V – Various	deferiprone	Ferriprox
H – Systemic hormonal preparations, excluding sex hormones and insulins	somatropin	NutropinaQ
N – Nervous system	levetiracetam	Keppra

Only three studies took into account the age classification according to the ICH/E11 guideline (one on Pedea and two on Aerius tablets), while the others considered different age groups.

Twenty-three studies included a classification of participants by gender, but no results by sex were reported.

3.3. Safety studies

A total of 105 safety studies were performed for 46 drugs and the total number of children included in the studies was 18153.

In 92 studies (88%), safety data were evaluated in short term within efficacy trials.

Four studies took into account the age classification according to the ICH/E11 guideline (two studies on Vfend and two on Aerius tablets), while the others considered different age groups.

Fifteen studies included a classification of participants by gender, but no results by sex were reported.

3.4. Compliance with ICH/E11 guideline

3.4.1. Timing and types of studies

The ICH/E11 guideline states that the timing and type of paediatric studies depend on the type of disease treated.

We therefore classified the diseases for which the 60 drugs are intended into the 3 groups (Table 4): 'predominantly or exclusively affecting paediatric patients' (Group 1), 'serious or life-threatening conditions occurring in both adult and paediatric

Table 4
Number (%) of studies conducted for the three disease groups

Disease	N of drugs to treat the disease	N (%) of drugs in PK studies	N (%) of drugs in efficacy studies	N (%) of drugs in safety studies
Predominantly or exclusively affecting paediatric patients (GROUP 1)	15	9 (60%)	14 (93.3%)	14 (93.3%)
Serious or life-threatening conditions occurring in both adult and paediatric patients, with no or limited therapeutic options (GROUP 2)	38	27 (73.7%)	31 (81.6%)	25(65.7%)
Other diseases or conditions (GROUP 3)	7	2 (28.6%)	4 (57.1%)	5 (71.4%)

patients, with no or limited therapeutic options' (Group 2) and 'other diseases or conditions' (Group 3).

Table 4 shows that in Group 1, 37% of the drugs had no PK study. Of these, for Cystagon a study is planned and for Nutropin previous PK studies were conducted for the same medicinal product. In the same category, only Neorecormon (Epoetin beta) lacks of efficacy and safety studies.

In Group 2 drugs have reached the commercialisation supported by a generally high number of studies, while in Group 3 a high percentage of safety studies was observed, as expected in accordance to the ICH/E11 guidance document.

3.4.2. Age classification

The ICH/E11 guideline states that when possible, extrapolation from adult or from older to younger patients may be appropriate for studies dealing with PK, efficacy and/or drug safety.

In the present analysis just 3 medicinal products were explicitly compliant:

- Pedea: CTs in pre-term, newborn and infants.
- Aerius tablets: CTs in adolescents (12–17 years).
- Vfend: CTs in children (2–11 years).

4. Conclusions

Our study found that, in the period 1995–2005, 60 drugs were licensed for use in children under the EMEA centralised procedure. These data show an increasing trend in the percentage of EMEA approved medicines for children compared with previously reported figures [1,6].

The majority of the studies concerns diseases predominantly or exclusively affecting paediatric patients and serious or life-threatening diseases, occurring in both adult and paediatric patients, for which there are currently no or limited therapeutic options. PK studies are performed for almost 70% of drugs when they are intended for these diseases. Efficacy and safety studies are carried out in more than 90% of the cases in drugs intended for diseases affecting children only and in more than 75% of the cases in drugs for life-threatening diseases.

The ICH/E11 guideline states that decisions on how to stratify studies and data by age need to consider development biology and pharmacology, and that sometimes it may be more appropriate to collect data over a broader age range and examine the effect of age as a continuous covariant. Our analysis found that few clinical studies were performed in compliance with the paediatric age groups as defined by the ICH/E11 guidelines. This is of particular concern especially when the adolescent age group is considered, since adolescents are frequently recruited together with adults.

The new Paediatric Regulation [4], in force from January 2007, is expected to dramatically change this situation.

Acknowledgements

This report is part of the Task-force in Europe for Drug Development for the Young (TEDDY) Network of Excellence supported by the European Commission's Sixth Framework Program (Contract n. 0005216 LSHBCT-2005-005126).

References

[1] A. Ceci, M. Felisi, M. Catapano, P. Baiardi, L. Cipollina, S. Ravera, S. Bagnulo, S. Reggio and G. Rondini, Medicines for children licensed by the European Agency for the Evaluation of Medicinal Products, *Eur J Clin Pharmacol* **58**(8) (2002 Nov), 495–500.

[2] S. Conroy, J. McIntyre, I. Choonara and T. Stephenson, Drug trials in children: problems and the way forward, *Br J Clin Pharmacol* **49**(2) (2000 Feb), 93–97. Review.

[3] European Parliament and the Council of the European Union, Directive 2001/20/EC of the European Parliament and of the Council of 4 April 2001 on the approximation of the laws, regulations and administrative provisions of the Member States relating to the implementation of good clinical practice in the conduct of clinical trials on medicinal products for human use, *Official Journal of the European Union* **L121** (2001), 34–44.

[4] European Parliament and Council Regulation (EC) No 1901/2006, 12 December 2006, on medicinal products for paediatric use and amending Regulation (EEC) No 1768/92, Directive 2001/20/EC, Directive 2001/83/EC and Regulation (EC) No 726/2004. *Official Journal of the European Union* **L378** (12.12.2006), 1–19.

[5] ICH Clinical Investigation of Medicinal Products in the Paediatric Population. ICH/Topic E11. *Eudralex* (2000).

[6] P. Impicciatore and I. Choonara, Status of new medicines approved by the European Medicines Evaluation Agency regarding paediatric use, *Br J. Clin Pharmacol* **48** (1999), 15–18.

Pharmaceuticals Policy and Law 11 (2009) 79–87
DOI 10.3233/PPL-2009-0208
IOS Press

Activity of Ethics Committees in Europe on issues related to clinical trials in paediatrics: Results of a survey

A. Altavilla[a], C. Giaquinto[b], D. Giocanti[c], C. Manfredi[d], J.-P. Aboulker[e], F. Bartoloni[f], E. Cattani[d], M. Lo Giudice[g], M.J. Mellado Peña[h], R. Nagler[i], C. Peterson[j], O. Vajnerova[k], F. Bonifazi[f] and A. Ceci[d,*]

[a]*Mediterranean University – Espace Ethique Méditerranéen, Bioethics Research Centre, Marseille, France*
[b]*Department of Paediatrics, University of Padova, Padova, Italy*
[c]*Mediterranean University – Division of Legal Medicine, Marseille, France*
[d]*Consorzio per Valutazioni Biologiche e Farmacologiche, Pavia, Italy*
[e]*Institut National de la Sante et Recherche Medicale, Villejuif, France*
[f]*I.RI.D.I.A. srl, Health Care Engineering, Bari, Italy*
[g]*Family paediatrician, AUSL 6 Palermo, Palermo, Italy*
[h]*Department of Paediatrics, Hospital Carlos III, Madrid, Spain*
[i]*Department of Oral and Maxillofacial Surgical and Oral Biochemistry Laboratory, Rambam Medical Center and Rappaport, Faculty of Medicine, Israel Institute of Technology-Technion, Haifa, Israel*
[j]*Department of Clinical Pharmacology, Linkopings Universitet, Linkopings, Sweden*
[k]*Department of Neurophysiology of Memory and Computational Neuroscience, Institute of Physiology, Academy of Sciences, Prague, Czech Republic*

The rights and well-being of children involved in clinical research in Europe should be assured by the respect of ethical considerations and legal rules. Specific provisions are included in the Directive 2001/20/EC (CT-Dir) aimed at providing a homogeneous ethical and legal context to perform clinical trials in Europe.

The TEDDY Network of Excellence carried out a "Survey on the ethical and legal frameworks existing in Europe for paediatric clinical trials" to examine the measures enforced by Member States to implement the CT-Dir and other relevant ethical norms.

The results showed that many differences exist in the protection of children enrolled in clinical trials. Such differences are especially due to a non-coordinated implementation of the Directive's Article 4 and a lack of public awareness on ethical issues in this field.

The recently approved 'Ethical considerations for clinical trials on medicinal products conducted with the paediatric population' should speed up the implementation of an 'ad hoc set of ethical rules' and increase the level of minors' protection. Nevertheless, in lack of 'binding rules', a coordination at European level is still needed. Public initiatives aiming at promoting in-depth debates have to be supported in order to encourage this process of coordination.

Keywords: TEDDY, ethics, paediatrics, clinical trials, informed consent, children assent

Abbreviations: Clinical Trial Directive or CT-Dir or CT Directive: Directive 2001/20/EC; EC: Ethics Committees; TEDDY: Task-force in Europe for Drug Development for the Young.

*Corresponding author: Adriana Ceci, Consorzio per Valutazioni Biologiche e Farmacologiche, Via Palestro, 26 – 27100 Pavia, Italy. Tel.: +39 0382 25075; Fax +39 0382 536544; E-mail: aceci@cvbf.net.

1. Introduction

Biomedical research should not be undertaken on human subjects without any account being taken of ethical guidelines and legal rules [12]. Special attention and specific guarantees are required for "vulnerable populations", as "children" [4], when these are involved in clinical research [9,13,14].

Currently, the rights and well-being of children participating in clinical research in Europe should be mainly assured by the respect of the EU Clinical Trials Directive's provisions [7]. The CT-Dir is a reference legislative instrument aimed at providing a homogeneous ethical, legal and scientific framework for the conduct of clinical trials in the European Union.

This Directive has been considered by the scientific community very differently: sometimes as necessary [20,21], sometimes as too bureaucratic [17] or simply harmful to the purpose of the development of clinical research [16]. Concerns have been expressed particularly when oncology or emergency settings are concerned [10,18].

The CT-Dir has included, for the first time in the European legislation context, some provisions with an ethical dimension, and in particular a specific article (Article 4) devoted to the protection of 'minors' and to the guarantee of their emotional, physiological and psychological specificities.

Nevertheless, since the Clinical Trial Directive makes reference to "ethical and scientific requirements" or soft law measures (e.g. good clinical practices, detailed guidance) it seems legitimate to fear that this reference to "non-binding rules" may be a source of confusion in applying "clear and harmonized ethical rules" in paediatric research across Europe.

Furthermore, as national authorities decide how principles set out in directives have to be incorporated into the National legislation in the light of Community objectives, the implementation process of CT-Dir might lead to some inequalities in the protection level of children involved in clinical trials across Europe.

In addition, provisions of the Clinical Trial Directive differ from those of other European/international ethical/legal sources such as the Oviedo Convention and its Additional Protocol (OC&AP), adopted by the Council of Europe [2,3]. This becomes evident if we consider the CT Directive provisions on the consent/assent procedure (with the respect of the children's will before being included -or their refusal to be included- as well as their withdrawal during the entire clinical research) and on the presence of paediatric expertises in Ethics Committees.

In February 2008, the European Commission released updated recommendations on ethical aspects of clinical trials involving children [5]. This document provides a new regulatory context, integrating principles contained in the Oviedo Convention, its Additional Protocol on biomedical research and in other relevant international ethical/legal sources, with the aim of insuring the protection of subjects involved in biomedical research while recognizing the importance of benefits derived from research. These Recommendations, integrating the CT Directive provisions, clarify the process of assessment of the benefit and risk balance, the process of information and consent/assent according to age groups and level of minors' maturity and the process of ethical review of paediatric protocols. They also deal with individual data protection and insurance issues. These Recommendations are expected to facilitate a coordinated approach to the application of the CT Directive across the EU, with special reference to paediatric research. In this context, it should be pointed out the importance of the Science and Society Action Plan of the European Commission [6], emphasizing the need for actions to raise awareness of ethical issues in science among researchers, when these issues are of direct interest to citizens (e.g. health, safety).

2. Aim of the study

TEDDY carried out a "Survey on the ethical and legal frameworks existing in Europe for paediatric clinical trials" to examine the measures enforced by Member States to implement Article 4 of the CT-Dir and other ethical norms relevant for clinical research in paediatrics.

The aim of this study was to refer on and disseminate among a large paediatric professional audience, the results of this investigation, integrating findings of a research work.

In the light of the recently adopted "Ethical considerations for clinical trials on medicinal products conducted with the paediatric population" [5], a description of the ethical and legal frameworks existing in the different European Countries to protect minors is provided.

2.1. Methodology

An *ad hoc* questionnaire was circulated among representatives of National Ethics Committees and other relevant National bodies (such as Health Ministries, Medicine Agencies and Research Councils) of 32 European Countries.

Issues covered by the Survey concerned:

- general initiatives (such as public debates or recommendations) taken to inform the public of clinical trials, with particular reference to paediatric issues;
- the Oviedo convention ratification, with particular reference to paediatric consent procedures;
- the legal/regulatory framework existing before the approval of the Directive 2001/20/EC;
- the legal/regulatory framework set up after Directive 2001/20/EC, with special reference to the implementation of Article 4 of this Directive;
- the existence of a minor's consent/assent procedure supporting the self-determination of the minor and his/her right to specific additional information;
- the existence of particular rules for the inclusion or withdrawal of children in clinical trials;
- the existence of Ethics Committees exclusively devoted to paediatric research as well as the guarantee of paediatric expertise in Ethics Committees.

3. Results

Until now, few data were available on the procedures followed by the different European Countries to implement the existing provisions with an ethical scope relevant for paediatric research and in particular, CT-Dir [1], Oviedo Convention [2] and more recently its Additional Protocol on Biomedical Research [3]. TEDDY Survey represents the first initiative aimed at evaluating the European ethical/legal framework for clinical trials in paediatrics.

Representatives of National Ethics Committees and other relevant National bodies in 27 European Countries participated in the Survey. Results are summarised in Table 1.

Table 2 shows the specific consent/assent procedure for minors that 6 Countries introduced in their National legislation.

Our results show that only 15 Countries provided an opinion/recommendation on Directive 2001/20/EC, only 7 provided an opinion/recommendation on clinical trials investigating medicinal products for paediatric use and only 6 Countries declared they organised initiatives aimed at debating issues related to clinical trials in paediatrics, as requested by the EC Science and Society Action Plan [6]. If all the States participating in the Survey (except Switzerland) implemented the CT-Directive, only 12 Countries (Cyprus, Czech Republic, Denmark, Estonia, Greece, Hungary, Iceland, Lithuania, Norway, Portugal, Slovakia and Spain) ratified the Oviedo Convention, by including in their internal laws the specific provisions on consent of minors involved in clinical researches provided by this Convention.

The majority of the Countries that participated in the Survey faithfully implemented the CT Directive provisions related to the inclusion criteria and consent procedures for minors (Article 4). Furthermore, 13 Countries declared that a framework for conducting paediatric clinical studies was already in place before the approval of the CT-Dir and 4 Countries have provided for an ethical reviewing process of clinical trials involving minors performed by specific Paediatric Ethics Committees.

However, in 6 Countries different approaches were followed in the implementation of Art. 4 of the CT-Directive, related to consent procedure.

Many Countries that ratified the Oviedo Convention, when implementing Directive 2001/20/EC, provide more restrictive rules aiming at protecting minors involved in clinical research. They assure more importance to the will of the minors (Spain) or consider their will necessary to involve them in clinical trials (Denmark, Estonia and the Netherlands). The expression of will is accepted at different age limits (12 years in Spain, 15–17 years in Denmark, 7–17 years in Estonia, 12 years in The Netherlands).

Even in the group of Countries that have not ratified the Oviedo Convention, specific paediatric guarantees are provided. This seems to occur more often in Countries where the debate on ethics has been appropriately developed before the entry into force of the Directive. So, in France it is provided that the consent of the minors prevails and it is impossible to pass over their refusal or the withdrawal of

Table 1
Results of the survey

COUNTRY	A	B	C	D	E	F	G
Austria	√	√					
Belgium		√					
Cyprus		√	√				
Czech Republic		√	√				
Denmark		√	√		√		15–17 years
Estonia	√	√	√		√		7–17 years
Finland	√	√		√	√	√	
France	√	√			√	√	
Germany	√	√			√	√	
Greece		√	√				
Hungary	√	√	√				
Iceland		√	√				
Ireland		√					
Italy	√	√		√			
Latvia		√					
Liechtenstein		√					
Lithuania	√	√	√				
Luxembourg		√					
Malta		√					
Netherlands	√	√		√	√		12 years
Norway	√	√	√				
Portugal		√	√				
Slovakia	√	√	√	√			
Sweden	√	√					
Spain	√	√	√		√		12 years
Switzerland				√			
United Kingdom		√					

A = PAEDIATRIC FRAMEWORK BEFORE CT-DIR; B = ART. 4 DIRECTIVE 2001/20/EC IMPLEMENTATION; C = OVIEDO CONVENTION (COE) RATIFICATION; D = ETHICS COMMITTEES (EC) DEVOTED TO MINORS; E = PAEDIATRIC CONSENT PROCEDURE DIFFERENT FROM DIRECTIVE PROVISIONS; F = SPECIFIC PROVISIONS ENSURING THE RESPECT OF MINOR'S REFUSAL OR WITHDRAWAL OF THEIR CONSENT TO PARTICIPATE IN A CLINICAL RESEARCH; G = SPECIFIC RULES ENSURING THAT MINOR'S OPINION SHOULD INCREASINGLY CARRY MORE WEIGHT IN THE FINAL DECISION. (THE AGE LIMITS TO FACILITATE THIS PROJECT).

their consent [19], while in Germany it is specified that "the minor should declare or express in any other way that he does not wish to take part in the clinical trial, this must be respected". Besides, "if the minor is in a position to comprehend the nature, significance and implications of the clinical trial and to form a rational intention in the light of these facts, then his consent shall also be required" [8]. Finnish legislation states that, taking into account the minor's age and maturity, his/her opinion opposing a research or a research measure shall be complied with. Furthermore, it specifies that the written consent of a minor having reached the age of 15 and capable of understanding the importance of the research procedure, shall

Table 2
Informed consent/assent procedures in respect of minors' will

COUNTRY	AGE LIMITS	SPECIFIC PROVISIONS ENSURING THE RESPECT OF THE CHILD'S WILL
Spain	12 years	If the minor is *12 years* of age or older, he/she *must also give his/her consent* to take part in the trial
Netherlands	12 years	If the minor is at least *12 years* old and if he/she can deemed capable of giving informed consent, it is prohibited to conduct trials without the *written consent of the subject* and the subject's parents (if they exercise parental responsibility or legal guardian)
Denmark	15–17 years	If the *15–17 year* old minor gives his/her informed consent, the holder of custody shall receive the same information and shall be involved in the decision of the 15–17 year old
Estonia	7–17 years	For a minor who is *7–17 years* old, to participate in a trial *the consent of the minor is necessary*
Finland	15 years	The *written consent of a minor*, that reached the *age of 15* and, in view of his/her age and maturity and the type of illness and research, is capable of understanding the importance of the research procedure, *shall be sufficient* to be involved in a research *if the research is likely to be of direct benefit to the minor's health*

be sufficient for him/her to be involved in a clinical trial, if this research is likely to be of direct benefit to his/her health. At the same time, the Finnish Advisory Board recommends that at any time the research subject or his/her guardian has the opportunity to request additional information about the research and his/her personal involvement.

With reference to paediatric expertise, only 4 Countries have set up an Ethics Committee specifically devoted to minors (Finland, Slovakia, The Netherlands and Italy). In the other Countries paediatric expertise is guaranteed mainly by inclusion of paediatric experts in Ethics Committees or by an advice from external experts, requested case by case especially when there is not a paediatrician in the Committee. In particular, in France this expertise is required only for minors under sixteen years [15], while in Denmark, paediatric expertise evaluation is not required in the case of non-interventional trials.

In The Netherlands, the legislation provides a special procedure for reviewing paediatric protocols: 'non therapeutic' *observational* clinical researches on minors are reviewed by an accredited Medical Ethics Review Committee (METC) working under the supervision of the Central Committee on Research Involving Human Subjects (CCMO); all non-therapeutic *intervention* researches on minors must undergo a medical ethics review by the CCMO.

4. Discussion and conclusions

The results of the TEDDY Survey demonstrate that many European Countries had paediatric measures in force before the approval of the Directive 20/2001/EC and that in the majority of cases, provisions in the paediatric field seem to have anticipated the measures undertaken by the Article 4 of the Directive, even if in a different manner.

The implementation of the Directive 2001/20/EC and of its Article 4 seemed to favour a gradual process of convergence in the legal measures towards a set of relevant "EU ethical values" for research on minors. Nevertheless, many differences related to the guarantees of children rights and to the ethical reviewing of paediatric protocols still exist. Thus, it seems legitimate to fear that these differences may lead to some inequalities in the protection of minors.

Such differences, in fact, seem to be of particular relevance if we consider the children's right to be clearly and adequately informed (according to their degree of maturity) before giving consent/assent and to freely refuse or withdraw from a trial. At this regard, the Survey demonstrated that few Countries developed a very high-level attention to the will of children, in contrast to other Countries that have no specific regulation on this point. Even the presence of Paediatric Ethics Committees and/or paediatric expertises in the Ethics Committees highlights different degrees of competence in reviewing clinical trials involving children. Thus, it seems legitimate to wonder if these differences have some effects on the safety of children and on the appropriateness of the clinical trials, especially if we consider that Ethics Committees are in charge of sensitive decisions related to selection criteria, end-points validation, adverse events to be collected, data protection, as well as rights, safety and well-being of human subjects involved in a trial.

The scarcity of high-level attention given to the respect of specific children's rights may depend mainly on the lack of coordination among different European ethical/legal documents [2,3,7] and ethical guidelines and norms. Furthermore, development of ethical debates at National and local level, in accordance with the European Commission's Science and Society Action Plan, may contribute to increase awareness of ethical issues related to paediatric research and to the full protection of children's rights. The percentage of legal instruments aimed at better protecting children involved in clinical trials, in fact, is higher in Countries where debates have been organised. In this sense, it could be interesting to note that the Finnish Advisory Board on Health Care Ethics (ETENE), in addition to other provisions, has recommended that 'the research subject or his/her guardian has the opportunity to request additional information about the research from the investigator and that varied and neutral information about the research must be available at any time'.

In conclusion, the results of the Survey conducted by TEDDY lead to several main considerations.

The CT Directive (Article 4) represents a real advancement to ensure a more protective ethical context for children involved in clinical trials.

The lack of coordination between different European ethical/legal sources [2,3, 7] generates some confusion in the implementation of Article 4 of the Directive at National level. The lack of public debates and initiatives aimed at increasing the social awareness have affected a homogenous high-level protection of children in all European Countries.

In the Recommendations [6] released by the European Commission in February 2008, many additional statements and some relevant clarifications have been provided, making reference to the main ethical/legal sources existing at European and international levels, in order to guarantee rights and health of subjects involved in biomedical research and taking into account the "vulnerability" of children.

It is TEDDY researchers' opinion that to promote the application of these updated rules, efforts are needed at both regulatory and scientific levels to increase public awareness of the ethical aspects of paediatric clinical trials and to identify adequate regulatory instrument for an efficacious coordination of such efforts.

Acknowledgements

This study is part of the Network of Excellence TEDDY (Task-force in Europe for the Drug Development for the Young) supported by the EC Sixth Framework Program (Contract n. 0005216 LSHBCT-2005-005126).

References

[1] A. Altavilla, C. Giaquinto and A. Ceci, European survey on ethical and legal framework of clinical trials in paediatrics: results and perspectives, *J Int Biœthique* **19(4)** (2008), in press.

[2] Council of Europe, Convention on Human Rights and Biomedicine, Strasbourg (1997). Entry into force in 1999.

[3] Council of Europe, Additional Protocol to the Convention on Human Rights and Biomedicine, concerning Biomedical Research, Strasbourg (2005). Entry into force in 2007.

[4] European Commission Enterprise Directorate General, Better Medicines for Children. Proposed regulatory actions on paediatric medicinal products, Consultation document, Brussels (2002).

[5] European Commission Enterprise Directorate General, Ethical considerations for clinical trials on medicinal products conducted with the paediatric population. Recommendations of the ad hoc group for the development of implementing guidelines for Directive 2001/20/EC relating to good clinical practice in the conduct of clinical trials on medicinal products for human use, available from URL http://ec.europa.eu/enterprise/pharmaceuticals/eudralex/homev10.htm (accessed 17 September 2008).

[6] European Commission, Science and Society in Europe, Action Plan, available from URL http://ec.europa.eu/research/science-society/action-plan/action-plan en. html (accessed 17 September 2008).

[7] European Parliament and the Council of the European Union, Directive 2001/20/EC of the European Parliament and of the Council of 4 April 2001 on the approximation of the laws, regulations and administrative provisions of the Member States relating to the implementation of good clinical practice in the conduct of clinical trials on medicinal products for human use, *OJ L 121* (2001), 34–44.

[8] Federal Republic of Germany, Arzneimittelgesetz – AMG – Medicinal Products Act (the Drug Law), as modified by the Article 12 of the Law of 14th August 2006, which entered into force on 18th August 2006, in: *Federal Law Gazette* I, p. 1869.

[9] D. Gill, F.P. Crawley, M. LoGiudice, S. Grosek, R. Kurz, M. de Lourdes-Levy, S. Mjönes, D. Nicolopoulos, A. Rubino, P.J. Sauer, M. Siimes, M. Weindig, M. Zach and T.L. Chambers; Ethics Working Group of the Confederation of European Specialists in Pediatrics, Guidelines for informed consent in biomedical research involving paediatric populations as research participants, *Eur J Pediatr* **162**(7–8) (2003), 455–458.

[10] R. Halila, Assessing the ethics of medical research in emergency settings: how do international regulations work in practice? *Sci Eng Ethics* **3**(3) (2007), 305–313.
[11] HMA. Heads of Medicines Agencies website, http://www.hma.eu (accessed 17 September 2008).
[12] C. Huriet, Introduction, in: *Ethical Eye: Biomedical research*, Council of Europe (2004) 17.
[13] J.E. John, The child's right to participate in research: myth or misconception? *Br J Nurs* **16**(3) (2007), 157–160.
[14] C.A. Knox and P.V. Burkhart, Issues related to children participating in clinical research, *J Pediatr Nurs* **22**(4) (2007), 310–318.
[15] Ministère de la santé et des solidarities, Décret n°2006-477 du 26 avril 2006 modifiant le chapitre Ier du titre II du livre Ier de la premère partie du code de la santé publique relatif aux recherches biomédicales (dispositions réglementaires). *Art. R 1123-4*, OJ 99 du 27 of April 2006
[16] C.D. Mitchell, Harmful impact of EU clinical trials directive: ... while paediatric oncology is being scuppered, *BMJ* **332**(7542) (2006), 666.
[17] M.J. Piccart, A. Goldhirsch, M.l Martin, J. Crown, R. Jakesz, H. Torbol Mouridsen, J. Bergh, J. G.M.Klijn, G. von Minckwitz, H. Roché and J. Jassem, European academics fight for the health of clinical trials, Rapid Responses, *BMJ* (2003 July 7).
[18] A. Plomer, Participation of children in clinical trials: UK, European and international legal perspectives on consent, *Med Law Int* **5**(1) (2000), 1–24.
[19] République Française. Loi n.2004-806 relative à la politique de santé publique of 9 August 2004. Art. L.1122-2-I-2. *OJ n.185* of 11 August 2004.
[20] A. Saint Raymond and D. Brasseur, Development of medicines for children in Europe: ethical implications, *Paediatr Respir Rev* **6**(1) (2005), 45–51.
[21] M.A. Weingarten, M. Paul and L. Leibovici, Assessing ethics of trials in systematic reviews, *BMJ* **328**(7446) (2004), 1013–1014.

Pharmaceuticals Policy and Law 11 (2009) 89–99
DOI 10.3233/PPL-2009-0204
IOS Press

Adverse drug reactions reporting in children

K. Verhamme[a], F. Bonifazi[b], A. Ceci[c,*], P. Elferink-Stinkens[a], M. Murray[d], A. Neubert[d], A. Nicolosi[e], B. Stricker[a], I. Wong[d] and M. Sturkenboom[a]

[a]*Pharmacoepidemiology Unit, Departments of Medical Informatics and Epidemiology & Biostatistics, Erasmus University Medical Center, Rotterdam, The Netherlands*
[b]*I.RI.D.I.A. srl, Health Care Engineering, Bari, Italy*
[c]*Consorzio per Valutazioni Biologiche e Farmacologiche, Pavia, Italy*
[d]*Centre for Paediatric Pharmacy Research, The School of Pharmacy and Institute of Child Health, University of London, London, UK*
[e]*Consiglio Nazionale delle Ricerche - Istituto di Tecnologie Biomediche, Milan, Italy*

The mission statement of the TEDDY project is to promote the research on the safe and effective use of drugs in children and to expand and integrate the knowledge and to build research capacity in the drug development for children.

One of the activities of WP1 – pharmacoepidemiology was to study the frequency and type of ADR reporting in children. For this analysis, we used data from the Uppsala Monitoring Centre (WHO collaborating Centre for International Drug Monitoring). All reports on ADRs in children (<18 years), sent to the monitoring centre between 2000 and 2004 were analysed.

This report contains the first results on the ADR reporting in children. Within this report, we mainly focus on the occurrence of ADRs with a fatal outcome. In further analysis, we will further explore the association between causal related deaths and the use of specific drugs.

Keywords: TEDDY, ADRs report, pharmacoepidemiology, children, WHO

1. Background

One of the objectives of TEDDY is to promote the research on safe and effective drugs in children.

Substantial research has been conducted on the safety of pharmaceutical products in adult patients but information on the safety of drugs in children is poor. In part, this relates to the fact that few clinical trials have been conducted in children. Pharmacokinetics and pharmacodynamics in children are different from adults and the combination with physiological development might place them at an increased risk of adverse drug reactions.

We wanted to study the frequency and the type of ADR reporting in children to get a better insight into the safety of drugs in this specific population group.

*Corresponding author: Adriana Ceci, Consorzio per Valutazioni Biologiche e Farmacologiche, Via Palestro 26, 27100 Pavia, Italy. Tel.: +39 0382 25075; Fax: +39 0382 536544; E-mail: aceci@ cvbf.net.

2. Methods

We used data from the Uppsala Monitoring Centre, WHO Collaborating Centre for International Drug Monitoring in Sweden. The WHO programme for International Drug Monitoring has been established in 1968 and as of 2007, 82 countries have joined the programme. The collaborating countries, forward the spontaneously reported cases of suspected ADRs to the WHO collaborating Centre. The case reports, recorded in a common format, are processed and stored in the ADR database [1]. The reports submitted to the Collaborating Centre in many instances describe no more than suspicions which have arisen from observation of an unexpected or unwanted event. In most instances, it cannot be proven that a pharmaceutical product or ingredient is the cause of the event. The reports, which are submitted to national centres, come from both regulatory and voluntary sources. Some national centres accept reports only from medical practitioners; other national centres accept reports from a wider spectrum of health professionals. Some national centres include reports from pharmaceutical companies in the information to the Collaborating Centre, other National Centres do not. It is thus obvious that the information is not homogeneous at least with respect to origin or likelihood that the pharmaceutical product caused the adverse reaction.

Within this database, we selected all ADRs reported in children ($<=$ 18 years) during the study period 1st January 2000 until 31st December 2004. Descriptive statistical analysis was used counting the ADRs according to the calendar year, the age and gender. We also studied the type of reported reaction terms and grouped them according to the highest frequency. For this analysis, we grouped reported terms both at the level of the system organ class and the preferred terms, all using WHO-art terminology. In addition, we studied the frequency of ADR reporting in relation to drug exposure. The drugs were classified according to the first level of the Anatomical Therapeutic Chemical (ATC) classification system. Finally, we focused on those ADRs with a fatal outcome and "definite" or "probable" causality if mentioned. Deaths were picked up by searching those reports that mentioned "died", "died – unrelated to reaction", "died – reaction may be contributory" as outcome. Deaths were classified as being causally related to the drug if the causality statement in the report was "definite" or "probable" or if "died – reaction may be contributory" was mentioned under the outcome. In this analysis we studied the frequency of fatal ADRs in relation to age, gender and drug exposure.

3. Results

Within the study period, 159171 reports were sent to the WHO Collaborating Centre. The mean numbers of ADRs per report and mean number of suspected drugs per report was 2.4 and 1.5 respectively. The reports mainly originated from the USA (55%) and the UK (11%) and the majority was spontaneously reported. 37% of the

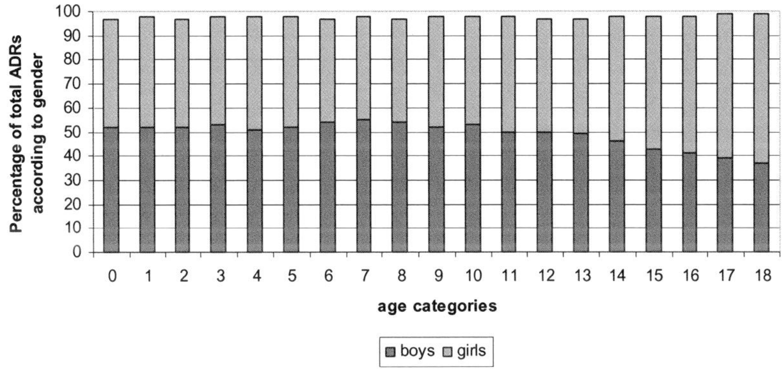

Fig. 1. Distribution of ADR reports according to gender for the different age categories.

Table 1
Number of ADR reports per age category

Age categories	Number of ADR reports in boys		Number of ADR reports in girls		Number of reports where gender is not mentioned		Total
	Number of reports	Percentage of total per age category	Number of reports	Percentage of total per age category	Number of reports	Percentage of total per age category	
0	18051	52	15554	45	918	3	34523
1	12904	52	11342	46	526	2	24772
2	3783	52	3228	45	198	3	7209
3	2885	53	2443	45	139	2	5467
4	4362	51	4042	47	179	2	8583
5	4406	52	3944	46	156	2	8506
6	2554	54	2013	43	117	2	4684
7	2184	55	1715	43	84	2	3983
8	2229	54	1793	43	100	2	4122
9	2465	52	2187	46	106	2	4758
10	2880	53	2487	45	93	2	5460
11	2987	50	2894	48	98	2	5979
12	2851	50	2692	47	207	4	5750
13	2360	49	2307	48	109	2	4776
14	2687	46	2981	52	109	2	5777
15	2723	43	3489	55	84	1	6296
16	2589	41	3609	57	108	2	6306
17	2396	39	3684	60	95	1	6175
18	2224	37	3737	62	83	1	6044
Total	79520	50	76141	48	3509	2	159170

reports were on children younger than 2 years. The number of reports was slightly higher in boys compared to girls especially for the younger age categories. As of the age of 14 years, the number of reported ADRs was higher in girls than in boys (Fig. 1 and Table 1).

The number of received ADRs per ATC category was the highest for vaccines –

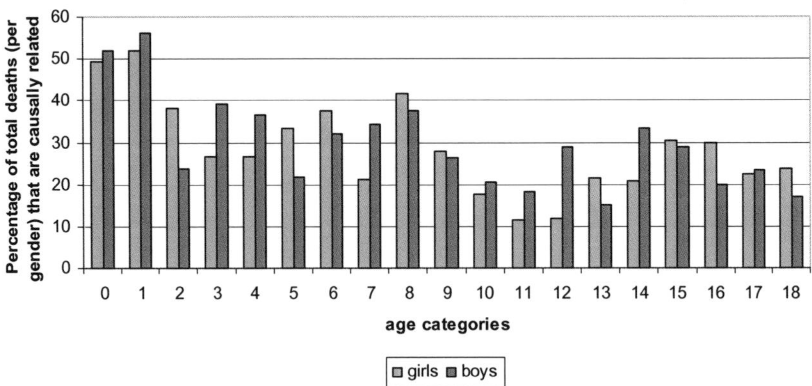

Fig. 2. Distribution of ADR reports according to gender for the different age categories.

approximately 70% of total ADRs that were received, had vaccines as suspected or interacting drug. The number of received ADRs per ATC category was also high for drugs for the nervous system (8%) and antimicrobial drugs excluding vaccines (7.5%). The distribution was rather similar between boys and girls apart from a somewhat higher number of ADRs that could be attributed to drugs for the nervous system in boys (8.8% in boys versus 6.9% in girls) and a higher number of ADRs that could be attributed to drugs for the genito-urinary system in girls (3.3% in girls versus 1.4% in boys) (Table 2).

2965 (1.9%) of the children died and for 1152 (39%) of these children, a potential association with the suspected drug could not be excluded. Fatal ADRs that were causally related were mainly reported in young children – up to 50% of deaths in children younger than 2 were causally related and this frequency was higher for boys than girls. The number of deaths that could be attributed to the use of drugs decreased with increasing age and no clear trend in gender differences could be observed (Table 3 and Fig. 2).

The rate of drug related deaths, expressed with the number of ADRs that had been received as denominator, was the highest for drugs given for haematological conditions namely 2.7%, followed by chemotherapy (1.5%) and drugs for the cardiovascular system (1.4%). These frequencies however, do not consider the actual drug use worldwide and the number of received ADRs might be low (Table 4). The rate of drug related deaths was consistently somewhat higher in boys than in girls, especially for the use of musculoskeletal agents and anti parasitic drugs.

The top 5 of reported reaction terms, among the children with causally related death were the following: apnoea (248 times reported), cardiac arrest (180), fever (136), respiratory disorder (107) and infection (100). The frequency of reported reaction terms amongst the causally related deaths are given in Table 5. Only those terms that occurred at least 10 times are provided in the table.

Table 2
Number of received ADRs per ATC code according to gender

ATC code	Females		Boys		Gender not specified		Total number of ADRs received	Percentage of total ADRs received
	Number of ADRs	Percentage of total ADRs received per gender	Number of ADRs	Percentage of total ADRs received per gender	Number of ADRs	Percentage of total ADRs received per gender		
A Alimentary tract and metabolism	3297	2.8	3128	2.5	206	4.4	6631	2.7
B Blood and blood forming organs	448	0.4	697	0.6	40	0.9	1185	0.5
C Cardiovascular system	951	0.8	1077	0.9	90	1.9	2118	0.9
D Dermatologicals	2477	2.1	2844	2.3	116	2.5	5437	2.2
G Genito urinary system and sex hormones	3803	3.3	1755	1.4	73	1.6	5631	2.3
H Systemic hormonal preparations, excluding sex hormones	525	0.5	701	0.6	28	0.6	1254	0.5
J General antiinfectives for systemic use, excluding vaccins	8447	7.3	9419	7.6	376	8.1	18242	7.5
J07 vaccins	81199	70.2	86071	69.5	2667	57.1	169937	69.6
L Antineoplastic and immunomodulating agents	2022	1.7	2230	1.8	130	2.8	4382	1.8
M Musculo-skeletal system	772	0.7	760	0.6	48	1.0	1580	0.6
N Nervous system	8037	6.9	10904	8.8	682	14.6	19623	8.0
P Antiparasitic products	372	0.3	262	0.2	10	0.2	644	0.3
R Respiratory system	2383	2.1	2930	2.4	171	3.7	5484	2.2
S Sensory organs	99	0.1	123	0.1	14	0.3	236	0.1
V Various	402	0.3	374	0.3	16	0.3	792	0.3
ATC code not specified	500	0.4	560	0.5	31	0.0	1091	0.4
Total	115734		123835		4698		244267	

Table 3
Number of deaths according to age category and gender

Age	Females			Boys			Gender not specified			Overall		
categories	Causally related death	% of causally related death for total number of deaths by age and gender	Total number of deaths	Causally related death	% of causally related death for total number of deaths by age and gender	Total number of deaths	Causally related death	% of causally related death for total number of deaths by age and gender	Total number of deaths	Causally related death	% of causally related death for total number of deaths by age and gender	Total number of deaths
0	265	49	536	404	52	779	13	20	66	682	49	1381
1	55	52	106	72	56	128	6	40	15	133	53	249
2	18	38	47	10	24	42	2	40	5	30	32	94
3	8	27	30	16	39	41	0	0	4	24	32	75
4	8	27	30	11	37	30	1	17	6	20	30	66
5	7	33	21	9	22	41	1	20	5	17	25	67
6	6	38	16	9	32	28	0	0	2	15	33	46
7	4	21	19	11	34	32	2	67	3	17	31	54
8	5	42	12	9	38	24	1	100	1	15	41	37
9	5	28	18	5	26	19	0	0	2	10	26	39
10	8	18	45	8	21	39	1	50	2	17	20	86
11	3	12	26	4	18	22	1	50	2	8	16	50
12	3	12	25	9	29	31	2	15	13	14	20	69
13	6	21	28	7	15	46	0	0	3	13	17	77
14	5	21	24	15	33	45	0	0	4	20	27	73
15	14	30	46	15	29	52	2	67	3	31	31	101
16	14	30	47	15	20	75	0	0	4	29	23	126
17	9	23	40	18	23	77	2	18	11	29	23	128
18	13	24	55	14	17	82	1	10	10	28	19	147
Total	456	39	1171	661	40	1633	35	22	161	1152	39	2965

Table 4
Number of ADRs with fatal outcome that were causally associated with the suspected ATC category

ATC code	Female			Male			Gender not specified			Total		
	Causally related death	Total number of ADRs received per ATC category	Causal death as % of number of ADRs received	Causally related death	Total number of ADRs received per ATC category	Causal death as % of number of ADRs received	Causally related death	Total number of ADRs received per ATC category	Causal death as % of number of ADRs received	Causally related death	Total number of ADRs received per ATC category	Causal death as % of number of ADRs received
A Alimentary tract and metabolism	16	3297	0.5	16	3128	0.5	6	206	2.9	38	6631	0.6
B Blood and blood forming organs	10	448	2.2	15	697	2.2	7	40	17.5	32	1185	2.7
C Cardiovascular system	11	951	1.2	16	1077	1.5	3	90	3.3	30	2118	1.4
D Dermatologicals	8	2477	0.3	15	2844	0.5	0	116	0.0	23	5437	0.4
G Genito urinary system and sex hormones	12	3803	0.3	9	1755	0.5	0	73	0.0	21	5631	0.4
H Systemic hormonal preparations, excluding sex hormones	5	525	1.0	10	701	1.4	1	28	3.6	16	1254	1.3
J General antiinfectives for systemic use, excluding vaccins	23	8447	0.3	25	9419	0.3	4	376	1.1	52	18242	0.3
J07 vaccins	792	81199	1.0	1193	86071	1.4	22	2667	0.8	2007	169937	1.2
L Antineoplastic and immunomodulating agents	26	2022	1.3	35	2230	1.6	4	130	3.1	65	4382	1.5
M Musculo-skeletal system	5	772	0.6	9	760	1.2	1	48	2.1	15	1580	0.9
N Nervous system	42	8037	0.5	67	10904	0.6	7	682	1.0	116	19623	0.6
P Antiparasitic products	3	372	0.8	4	262	1.5	0	10	0.0	7	644	1.1
R Respiratory system	21	2383	0.9	30	2930	1.0	0	171	0.0	51	5484	0.9
S Sensory organs	0	99	0.0	0	123	0.0	0	14	0.0	0	236	0.0
V Various	0	402	0.0	1	374	0.3	1	16	6.3	2	792	0.3
ATC code not specified	1	500	0.2	0	560	0.0	0	31	0.0	1	1091	0.1
Total	975	115734	0.8	1445	123835	1.2	56	4698	1.2	2476	244267	1.0

Table 5
Frequency of reported ADR terms in children with causally related death (only frequencies of 10 or more have been selected)

ADR Term	Number	Percentage of total number of ADRs in children with causally related death
APNOEA	248	6.6%
CARDIAC ARREST	227	6.0%
FEVER	151	4.0%
RESPIRATORY DISORDER	107	2.8%
INFECTION	100	2.7%
AGITATION	98	2.6%
PNEUMONIA	81	2.1%
CYANOSIS	80	2.1%
PURPURA	80	2.1%
PULMONARY OEDEMA	74	2.0%
CONVULSIONS	70	1.9%
STUPOR	62	1.6%
HAEMORRHAGE NOS	60	1.6%
DYSPNOEA	57	1.5%
ENCEPHALOPATHY	46	1.2%
COMA	42	1.1%
OEDEMA CEREBRAL	39	1.0%
CIRCULATORY FAILURE	37	1.0%
VOMITING	37	1.0%
DIARRHOEA	32	0.8%
SEPSIS	31	0.8%
ANOREXIA	30	0.8%
CRYING ABNORMAL	30	0.8%
HYPOTONIA	28	0.7%
SOMNOLENCE	28	0.7%
HEART DISORDER	26	0.7%
SUICIDE ATTEMPT	26	0.7%
CARDIAC FAILURE	24	0.6%
HYPOXIA	24	0.6%
MENINGITIS	24	0.6%
ATELECTASIS	23	0.6%
BRONCHITIS	21	0.6%
CONDITION AGGRAVATED	21	0.6%
ASPHYXIA	20	0.5%
CARDIOMYOPATHY	20	0.5%
CONGENITAL ANOMALY NOS	19	0.5%
RASH	19	0.5%
DEHYDRATION	18	0.5%
RHINITIS	18	0.5%
LYMPHADENOPATHY	17	0.5%
RESPIRATORY DEPRESSION	17	0.5%
ENCEPHALOMYELITIS	16	0.4%
HEPATIC FAILURE	16	0.4%
PHARYNGITIS	16	0.4%
ACIDOSIS	15	0.4%
BRADYCARDIA	15	0.4%
MULTIPLE ORGAN FAILURE	15	0.4%

Table 5, continued

ADR Term	Number	Percentage of total number of ADRs in children with causally related death
PALLOR	15	0.4%
PULMONARY HAEMORRHAGE	15	0.4%
CEREBROVASCULAR DISORDER	14	0.4%
HYPERTONIA	13	0.3%
OEDEMA	13	0.3%
COUGHING	12	0.3%
GASTROENTERITIS	12	0.3%
HEPATOCELLULAR DAMAGE	12	0.3%
ANAPHYLACTIC SHOCK	11	0.3%
CSF ABNORMAL	11	0.3%
MEDICATION ERROR	11	0.3%
NEOPLASM NOS	11	0.3%
RIGORS	11	0.3%
ARRHYTHMIA	10	0.3%
HYPERTENSION PULMONARY	10	0.3%
HYPOTHERMIA	10	0.3%
INJECTION SITE REACTION	10	0.3%
LIVER FATTY	10	0.3%
RENAL FUNCTION ABNORMAL	10	0.3%

4. Conclusions

The number of ADR reports in children that are sent to the WHO is substantial and in 0.7% of these reports death was recorded as potentially causally related, which merits further attention. Reporting bias however, could highly influence the estimates in this hypothesis-generating-study and this should be taken into account when interpreting the data. In addition, it should be emphasized that we did not have information on the actual consumption of the drugs in the pediatric population. One could well imagine that drugs often used in children, such as vaccines, might generate more ADRs. Finally, our definition of fatal ADRs did not include "death" as reported term itself or when only indicated in a serious criteria field, meaning that we will probable have underestimated the number of drugs with fatal outcome. Despite these limitations, we believe that analysing data from spontaneous ADR reporting might be helpful to prioritize studies on safety of certain drugs in children.

Acknowledgements

This report is part of the Task-force in Europe for Drug Development for the Young (TEDDY) Network of Excellence supported by the European Commission's Sixth Framework Program (Contract n. 0005216 LSHBCT-2005-005126).

We thank the WHO Collaborating Centre for International Drug Monitoring in Sweden for providing the data on ADR reporting in children. The authors want to emphasize that the information in the report does not represent the opinion of the WHO. A general statement from the WHO regarding release of data from the WHO Collaborating Centre is attached (Appendix 1).

Reference

[1] I.R. Edward and S. Ollson, WHO programme-global monitoring, in: *Pharmacovigilance,* R.D. Mann and E.B. Andrews, eds, Wiley, London, 2002, pp. 169–182.

Appendix 1

WHO Collaborating Centre
for International Drug Monitoring
Stora Torget 3, S-753 20 Uppsala, Sweden

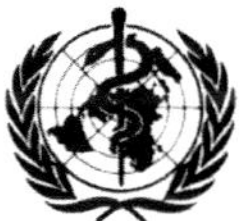

Tel: +46-18-65 60 60
Fax: +46-18-65 60 80
E-mail: info@who-umc.org

CAVEAT DOCUMENT

Accompanying statement to data released from the WHO Collaborating Centre

The WHO Collaborating Centre for International Drug Monitoring, Uppsala, Sweden receives summary clinical reports about individual suspected adverse reactions to pharmaceutical products from National Centres in countries participating in a Collaborative Programme. Only limited details about each suspected adverse reaction are received at the Centre. It is important that the limitations and qualifications which apply to the information and its use are understood.

The term "pharmaceutical product" is used instead of "drug" to emphasize that products marketed under one generic or trade name may vary in their content of active or other ingredients, both in time or from place to place.

The reports submitted to the Collaborating Centre in many instances describe no more than suspicions which have arisen from observation of an unexpected or unwanted event. In most instances it cannot be proven that a pharmaceutical product or ingredient is the cause of an event.

The reports, which are submitted to National Centres, come from both regulatory and voluntary sources. Some national Centres accept reports only from medical practitioners; other National Centres accept reports from a wider spectrum of health professionals. Some National Centres include reports from pharmaceutical companies in the information submitted to the Collaborating Centre; other National Centres do not.

The volume of reports for a particular pharmaceutical product may be influenced by the extent of use of the product, publicity, nature of reactions and other factors which vary over time, from product to product and country to country. Moreover, no information is provided on the number of patients exposed to the product.

Thus the sources of reports accepted by National Centres vary, as do the proportions.

A number of National Centres which contribute information to the Collaborating Centre make an assessment of the likelihood that a pharmaceutical product caused the suspected reaction. Other National Centres do not document such assessments on individual reports in the WHO data base.

Processing time varies from country to country. Reporting figures obtained from the Collaborating Centre may therefore differ from those obtained directly from National Centres.

For the above reasons interpretations of adverse reaction data, and particularly those based on comparisons between pharmaceutical products, may be misleading. The information tabulated in the accompanying printouts is not homogeneous with respect to the sources of the information or the likelihood that the pharmaceutical product caused the suspected adverse reaction. Some describe such information as "raw data". Any use of this information must take into account at least the above.

Some National Centres which have authorized release of their information strongly recommend that anyone who intends to use it should contact them for interpretation.

Any publication, in whole or in part, of the obtained information must have published with it a statement:

(i) of the source of the information,

(ii) that the information is not homogeneous at least with respect to origin or likelihood that the pharmaceutical product caused the adverse reaction,

(iii) that the information does not represent the opinion of the World Health Organization.

Omission of these 3 statements may exclude the responsible person or organization from further information from the system.

Pharmaceuticals Policy and Law 11 (2009) 101–109
DOI 10.3233/PPL-2009-0215
IOS Press

Availability of medicines for rare diseases in EU Countries

Annalisa Trama[a], Daniela Pierannunzio[a], Alberto Loizzo[a], Domenica Taruscio[a] and A. Ceci[b,*]
[a]*National Centre for Rare Diseases, Istituto Superiore di Sanità, Roma, Italy*
[b]*Consorzio per Valutazioni Biologiche e Farmacologiche, Pavia, Italy*

The European Medicines Agency has expressed 50 positive opinions recommending the granting of a marketing authorisation for an orphan medicinal product since the Regulation on orphan medicinal products (OMPs) entered into force in 2000. However, OMPs authorised at EU level are not always available at Member States (MS) level. We developed and distributed a questionnaire to collect information on the availability of 20 OMPs authorised before October 2006. The questionnaire included questions on the date of national market availability; the possibility of pre-marketing access programme; the distribution channel, the availability of a reimbursement policy. Twelve MS provided information: Austria, Belgium, Czech Republic, Denmark, Estonia, Finland, Hungary, Ireland, Italy, Latvia, Slovakia and UK. Results demonstrate that the availability of OMPs varies greatly among the 12 MS considered and market availability delays are highly variable. OMPs are often expensive drugs and the different MS reimbursement policies are hindering access to OMPs. Data show that since 2000 the number of OMPs has increased however issues including costs and reimbursement policies at MS level represent major barriers to real OMPs accessibility. This is a critical situation that deserves attention because of the evident inequalities that do exist with regards to OMPs accessibility among MS.

Keywords: TEDDY, orphan medicinal product, accessibility, availability

1. Introduction

Medicines for rare diseases also called ‘orphan’ medicinal products are those medicines intended for the diagnosis, prevention or treatment of life-threatening or chronically debilitating conditions that affect no more than five in 10,000 people in the European Union, or are medicines which, for economic reasons, would be unlikely to be developed without incentives [3].

The EU legislative framework [9] introducing an EU public health policy on orphan medicinal products (OMPs) came into effect in the European Union in April 2000 with the aim of stimulating research and development of medicinal products for rare diseases by providing incentives to the pharmaceutical industry. Applications for designation of orphan medicines are reviewed by the European Medicines Agency (EMEA) through the Committee for Orphan Medicinal Products (COMP). This

*Corresponding author: Adriana Ceci, Consorzio per Valutazioni Biologiche e Farmacologiche, Via Palestro, 26–27100 Pavia, Italy. Tel.: +39 0382 25075; Fax +39 0382 536544; E-mail: aceci@cvbf.net.

initiative helps to give patients suffering from rare diseases access to the same quality of treatment as other patients.

The OMPs designated to date cover a wide variety of rare diseases, including genetic diseases and rare cancers, for most of which there are either no or only unsatisfactory treatment options. A large number of these diseases affect children and newborn babies.

The status of orphan applications follow (update November 2008) [4]:

- a total of 873 applications have been submitted for the designation of OMPs;
- the COMP has adopted 598 positive opinions on orphan designation;
- a total of 569 medicines have been awarded orphan-designation status by the European Commission;
- a total of 218 applications have been withdrawn and 13 received a negative COMP opinion;
- a total of 50 medicines have received both an orphan designation and a Community marketing authorisation.

In this context, this article aims at providing an overview of the availability of OMPs in EU Member States and at describing major challenges limiting the access to OMPs.

2. Methodology

A questionnaire was developed in collaboration with the European Organisation for Rare Diseases (EURORDIS): a patient-driven alliance of patient organisations and individuals active in the field of rare diseases. The questionnaire aimed at assessing the OMPs' availability in EU Countries. Twenty OMPs authorized by EMEA before October 2006 were considered for this study and the list is reported in Table 1. The questionnaire included the following items:

- ATC code;
- date of national market availability;
- possibility of pre-marketing access programme in Country;
- distribution channel (pharmacy/hospital);
- reimbursement provided by insurance company or public agency and reimbursement rate (%).

The questionnaire was distributed to the Responsible of the Ministry of Health or to the National Drug Agencies of the 25 EU Countries and to all the partners of the Network of Public Health Institution on Rare Diseases (NEPHIRD). NEPHIRD is a project supported by the European Commission (http://ec.europa.eu/health/ph_threats/non_com/rare_3_en.htm) for a 4-year period (November 2002-2006) coordinated by the National Centre for Rare Diseases (Istituto Superiore di Sanità – Italy, http://www.iss.it/cnmr/neph/index.php?lang=2).

Table 1
List of orphan medicinal products considered in the survey

Trade name	Product	Designated orphan indication
Aldurazyme	Laronidase	Mucopolysaccharidosis, type I
Busilvex	Busulfan	Conditioning treatment prior to hematopoietic progenitor cell transplantation
Carbaglu	N-carbamyl-L-glutamic acid	Treatment of N-acetylglutamate synthetase (NAGS) deficiency
Fabrazyme	Alpha-Galactosidase A	Treatment of Fabry disease
Glivec	Imatinib mesylate	Treatment of chronic myeloid leukaemia
Onsenal	Celecoxib	Treatment of Familial Adenomatous Polyposis
Replagal	Alpha-Galactosidase A	Treatment of Fabry disease
Somavert	Pegvisomant	Treatment of acromegaly
Tracleer	Bosentan	Treatment of pulmonary arterial hypertension and chronic thromboembolic pulmonary hypertension
Trisenox	Arsenic trioxide	Treatment of acute promyelocytic leukaemia
Ventavis	Iloprost	Treatment of primary and of the following forms of secondary pulmonary hypertension: connective tissue disease pulmonary hypertension, drug-induced pulmonary hypertension, portopulmonary hypertension, pulmonary hypertension associated with congenital heart disease, chronic thromboembolic pulmonary hypertension
Zavesca	1,5-(Butylimino)-1,5-dideoxy, D-glucitol	Treatment of Gaucher Disease
Litak	Cladribine (subcutaneous use)	Treatment of indolent non-Hodgkin's lymphoma
Lysodren	Mitotane	Treatment of adrenal cortical carcinoma
Orfadin	Nitisinone	Treatment of tyrosinaemia type I
Pedea	Ibuprofen	Treatment of patent ductus arteriosus
Photobarr	Porfimer sodium (for use with photodynamic therapy)	Treatment of high-grade dysplasia in Barrett's Esophagus
Prialt	Ziconotide (intraspinal use)	Treatment of chronic pain requiring intraspinal analgesia
Xagrid	Anagrelide Hydrochloride	Treatment of essential thrombocythaemia
Wilzin	Zinc acetate dihydrate	Treatment of Wilson's disease

Source: EMEA register of designated Orphan Medicinal Products.

In addition, to ensure the quality of the information collected, the COMP members were requested to personally fill in or to direct the questionnaire to the most appropriate person.

The questionnaire was circulated and continuous follow up was ensured by e-mail between March 2006 and July 2006.

3. Results

Twelve out of 25 contacted countries sent back the questionnaire filled in. Of the non respondents: 4 ensured an answer within a short time (however information were not provided regardless the reminder sent); 4 did not receive/read the mail (no confirmation was sent back) and others received the e-mail but did not provide any answer.

The countries that filled in the questionnaire follow: Austria, Belgium, Czech Republic, Denmark, Estonia, Finland, Hungary, Ireland, Italy, Latvia, Slovakia and UK.

The list of OMPs available for each country (at July 2006) is reported in Table 2.

A brief summary of the main findings for each country follow.

Austria: all the 20 drugs in the list were available in country. No further information were provided.

Belgium: 15 out of the 20 OMPs listed were available and were authorized from 2002 to 2006.

Czech Republic: 14 out of the 20 OMPs listed were available and directly distributed by the pharmacies (even in hospitals OMPs are distributed through the hospital pharmacy). OMPs are subject to special reimbursement regime (i.e. requiring consent of a designated medical insurance company with doctor who audits drug expenses). Only for 1 OMP (Aldurazyme) there was an insurance coverage of 100%. There isn't a pre-marketing access programme for any of the products.

Denmark: 15 out of the 20 OMPs listed were available and authorized from November 2001 to March 2005. No pre-marketing access programme is available; however, it is possible to get a compassionate use permit for medicinal products not authorised in Denmark. There is no reimbursement for medicinal products distributed exclusively from the hospitals as in this case the drugs are provided for free (all OMPs on the list were restricted to hospital distribution).

Estonia: 4 of the 20 OMPs listed were available and were authorised between 2002 and 2006. Three (Busilvex, Fabrazyme and Glivec) out of the 4 were 100% reimbursed while 1 (Onsenal) was 50% reimbursed. Information on pre-marketing access programme and distribution channel were not provided.

Finland: 11 out the 20 OMPs listed were available in Finland. Data about the starting date of availability were not provided.

Hungary: 6 out of 20 OMPs listed were available. Three products of the list (Replagal, Tracleer and Ventavis) were registered in Hungary without an orphan drug status. They were registered since 2002 (the last one being registered in 2006). No pre-marketing access programme is available; for 2 (Fabrazyme and Zavesca) out of the 3 OMPs registered with the orphan drugs status there was no reimbursement, while for the third one (Glivec) the reimbursed rate was 100%.

Ireland: 6 out of the 20 OMPs listed were available in Ireland and were authorized from 2002 to 2005.

Italy: 16 out the 20 OMPs listed were available and were authorized from November 2004 to August 2005; pre-marketing access programme is available for those OMPs not yet authorized. All OMPs are distributed only from the hospitals and are 100% reimbursed.

Latvia: only 3 of the 20 OMPs listed were available in Latvia; 1 (Glivec) of them was authorized in 2005 and the remaining 2 (Somavert and Tracleer) in 2006.

Table 2
Orphan medicinal products available per country (July, 2006)

	Austria	Belgium	Czech Republic	Denmark	Estonia	Finland	Hungary	Ireland	Italy	Latvia	Slovakia	UK
Aldurazyme	×	×	×	×		×			×		×	×
Busilvex	×		×	×	×				×		×	×
Carbaglu	×	×		×					×		×	×
Fabrazyme	×	×	×	×	×	×	×		×		×	×
Glivec	×	×	×	×	×	×	×	×	×	×	×	×
Litak	×	×	×	×		×			×		×	×
Lysodren	×	×	×	×		×			×		×	×
Onsenal	×		×		×							
Orfadin	×	×		×		×					×	×
Pedea	×	×	×	×					×			×
Photobarr	×											
Prialt	×											×
Replagal	×	×	×	×			×		×			×
Somavert	×	×	×	×		×		×	×	×	×	×
Tracleer	×	×	×	×		×	×	×	×	×		×
Trisenox	×	×	×						×		×	×
Ventavis	×		×	×		×	×	×	×		×	×
Wilzin	×	×							×			×
Xagrid	×	×		×		×		×	×			×
Zavesca	×	×	×	×		×	×	×	×			×

Source: our elaboration.

Table 3
Information on number of countries where OMPs are available, first year of availability, distribution channel and reimbursement

OMP trade name	Number of countries where OMP is available	Ranges of first availability	Number of countries where OMPs are distributed by pharmacies	Number of countries where OMPs are 100% reimbursed
Aldurazyme	5	2003–2004	2	4
Busilvex	6	2002–2005	1	4
Carbaglu	4	2002–2006	0	2
Fabrazyme	7	2001–2006	2	5
Glivec	7	2001–2006	2	6
Onsenal	2	2002	1	3
Replagal	4	2001	2	2
Somavert	5	2002–2004	1	3
Tracleer	5	2002–2003	1	3
Trisenox	3	2002	1	2
Ventavis	6	2003–2004	2	3
Zavesca	5	2003–2005	1	3
Litak	4	2004	1	3
Lysodren	4	2004–2005	1	4
Orfadin	3	2005	1	1
Pedea	3	2004	1	1
Photobarr	0	not available	not available	not available
Prialt	0	not available	not available	not available
Xagrid	2	2005	1	1
Wilzin	2	2004–2005	0	2

Source: our elaboration.

Slovakia: 11 out the 20 OMPs listed were available in the market; they were authorized from August 2001 to February 2005. For 2 OMPs there was a pre-marketing access programme; all of them were distributed through hospitals and are 100% reimbursed. Only one (Ventavis) was distributed through pharmacies.

UK: 18 out of the 20 OMPs listed were available in UK; they were authorised between August 2001 and January 2006. Most OMPs were distributed through hospitals and some of them through both hospitals and pharmacies. While there is no official pre-marketing access programme, in general, physicians are able to prescribe medicines procured via importers, if they are not marketed in the UK.

Information on number of countries where OMPs are available, first year of availability, distribution channel and reimbursement rate are summarised in Table 3.

Accordingly to our survey, out of the 20 OMPs having received a market authorization in the EU only 1 (Glivec) was available in all the 12 countries considered in the study. In only 1 country (Austria) all the 20 OMPs were available.

OMPs were mainly distributed through hospitals, less frequently through pharmacies.

Each Ministry of Health or National Drug Agency negotiates prices separately with the pharmaceutical companies. Sponsor tends to start negotiating with Member States that grant them a higher price in order to use it as a benchmark in their negotiations with other countries.

The date of national market availability was not reported by several countries, which usually reported only the year of first availability. Because of this, it was not possible to assess whether the legal delay limit for placing medicinal products on the EU market, which is 180 days starting from the authorization by EMEA [10], was observed. However, according to few examples provided in the questionnaire, it seems that this rule is not often observed: Fabrazyme and Glivec were authorised by EMEA in 2001 but they were available in some countries 5 years later, in 2006.

4. Discussion

Our results demonstrate that the availability of OMPs varies greatly among the 12 EU MS considered and that market availability delays are highly variable. These results are confirmed by additional surveys undertaken by EURORDIS [5,6].

According to the most recent EURORDIS survey [7], the countries with most OMPs available to patients (20 or 21 OMPs) are Finland, France, Germany, and Sweden. In Austria, Czech Republic, Denmark, Italy, Netherlands, Norway, Spain, Switzerland and United Kingdom there are 15 to 19 OMPs available. The worst contenders are Iceland, Latvia and Lithuania with only up to 4 OMPs available.

Our results reveal that country policies on OMPs differ among EU MS. This is again confirmed by EURORDIS surveys [7], concluding that OMPs are often fully reimbursed to patients however patients from Hungary, Spain and the United Kingdom have to pay up to 94% of that price for the same drugs, and by the Alcimed study [1]. In Hungary few OMPs (Glivec, Fabrazyme, Replagal) are 100% reimbursed; others (Aldurazyme, Revatio, Exjade, Somavert, Lysodren, Tracleer, Myozyme, Orfadin) are available for individual reimbursement. In Italy, all OMPs are fully charged to the national health care service [8].

Another important issue revealed by our survey is the delay in availability of OMPs and EURORDIS confirms that the 180 day legal delay for placing medicinal products on the market was still not respected in 2007.

5. Conclusions

The EMEA has expressed 50 positive opinions recommending the granting of a marketing authorisation for an OMP by the European Commission since the Regulation on orphan medicinal products entered into force in 2000. OMPs covering more than 30 conditions and potentially benefiting some 1.6 million patients have been made available for use in the European Union since 2001.

The success of the Regulation on OMPs is linked to the work of the Committee for Orphan Medicinal Products (COMP), the EMEA's scientific committee in charge of reviewing applications for designation of medicinal products as orphan medicines.

However, OMPs authorised at EU level are not always available at MS level leaving patients without the chance to get the treatment for their life threatening diseases (the OMPs availability is extremely heterogeneous). The market availability delay of OMPs is high and highly variable among MS with countries with a small population suffering from a longer delay in availability of OMPs.

In addition, OMPs are often expensive drugs and the different MS policies on OMPs reimbursement are hindering access to OMPs. Also in countries with high GDP only a small number of OMPs are really available.

These data show that since 2000 the number of OMPs has increased, however different issues including costs and/or reimbursement policy at MS level represent major barriers to real OMPs accessibility to patient.

This is a critical situation that deserves urgent attention because of the evident inequalities that do exist with regards to OMPs accessibility among MS.

As reported also in the Commission communication on Rare Diseases: Europe's challenge [2], a solution to this situation should be found in order to ensure equal access to orphan drugs throughout the EU.

If the EU Commission has a major role to play, including a wider engagement of MS, MS Competent Authorities and pharmaceutical companies, many additional initiatives should be promoted to contribute to ensuring that all patients with rare disease have access to the OMPs available for their diseases [2,11]:

1. increase awareness on rare diseases and orphan drugs to ensure political and general public support for rare disease patients;
2. communicate better the potential impact of rare disease research outcomes in the understanding of common disease pathways;
3. promote fiscal measures to stimulate the interest of pharma industries, in particular those with high level of innovation, in research and development for orphan drugs;
4. identify mechanism for ensuring that pharma industries receiving orphan designation and centralised marketing authorisation will register their products in all countries including the smaller EU countries;
5. boost the public financing of independent research;
6. promote the assessment of the therapeutic added value of orphan drugs at European level, to accelerate negotiation phase at national level;
7. strengthen international collaboration;
8. support an early dialogue between companies and authorities;
9. encourage transparency on orphan drugs price;
10. promote reimbursement policies able to ensure access to orphan drugs for all patients.

Acknowledgements

This study is part of the Network of Excellence TEDDY (Task-force in Europe for the Drug Development for the Young) supported by the EC Sixth Framework

Program (Contract n. 0005216 LSHBCT- 2005-005126).

References

[1] Alcimed, Study on Orphan drugs, Overview of the conditions for marketing orphan drugs in Europe. Available at URL: http://ec.europa.eu/enterprise/pharmaceuticals/orphanmp/doc/pricestudy/final final_report_part_1_web.pdf, Accessed 20 November 2008.
[2] Commission of the European Communities. Communication from the Commission to the European Parliament, the Council, the European Economic and Social Committee and the Committee of the Regions on rare diseases: Europe's challenges, COM(2008) 679 final (11.11.2008) Available at URL: http://ec.europa.eu/health/ph_threats/non_com/rare_10_en.htm. Accessed 21 November 2008
[3] European Medicines Agency (EMEA). Human medicines - Orphan medicinal products. Available at URL: http://www.emea.europa.eu/htms/human/orphans/intro.htm. Accessed 20 November 2008.
[4] European Medicines Agency (EMEA), List of orphan-designated authorised medicines, EMEA/ 563575/2008 (6 November 2008).
[5] European Organisation for Rare Diseases (Eurordis), Survey of orphan drugs availability in Europe, 2002, Available at URL: http://www.eurordis.org, Accessed 20 November 2008.
[6] European Organisation for Rare Diseases (Eurordis), Survey of orphan drugs availability in Europe, 2004. Available at URL: http://www.eurordis.org, Accessed 20 November 2008.
[7] European Organisation for Rare Diseases (Eurordis), Survey of orphan drugs availability in Europe, 2007, Available at URL: http://www.eurordis.org, Accessed 20 November 2008.
[8] European Organisation for Rare Diseases (Eurordis), Round Table of Companies "Do rare diseases patients have real access to orphan drugs in Europe?", July 9th, 2007 - Barcelona, Spain.
[9] European Parliament and Council Regulation 141/2000/EC, 16 December 1999 on Orphan Medicinal Products, *Official Journal of the European Communities* **L18** (22.01.2000), 1–5.
[10] Council of the European Communities. Council Directive 89/105/EEC of 21 December 1988 relating to the transparency of measures regulating the pricing of medicinal I products for human use and their inclusion in the scope of national health insurance systems, *Official Journal of the European Communities* **L40** (11.2.1989), 8.
[11] F. Meyer, Timely and equitable access to orphan medicines across Member States, The European HAS workshop November 2006, Paris in report of the 4th European Conference on rare diseases, Patients at the heart of rare diseases policy development, Lisbon, 2007, 141–143.